FORWARD

This book started in 1974 – at least, the idea did. I actually started working on it around 1980, when I realized what tremendous human interest I had the opportunity to watch. I wasn't sure how it would turn out, if at all, but, then again, you're reading it!

The book is a mix of what it takes to be a Paramedic, what they see through the lens of their own eyes and the thoughts, smells and feelings on what takes place on the streets of this country every day.

EMTs and Paramedics <u>are</u> the gates keepers of the medical profession. Before the GP gets to see the family member, before the ER (emergency room) charts one symptom, before the surgeon makes one cut, EMS personnel evaluate and treat millions of patients, most in darkened hallways or overturned cars, some under fire and many under other horrific conditions.

They do so with a smile in their heart and a caring that most cannot comprehend. Many are volunteers, leaving their families and warm dinner to head out to someone who is having a baby or battling cancer. They do so without hope of compensation and with a hope that someday, someone will do the same for them. In the country of givers, they are at the top of the list.

Others are paid and work for an organization whose role is to help those who are having a terrible day or moment in their life. They are no less a hero because they are paid but, simply hold a different performance.

Regardless of paid, or volunteer, the stories inside are a collection of 40 years of helping people at their lowest times – of caring for someone when caring was all that was needed and doing lifesaving skills when caring wasn't enough. You will also find stories of people in my life, many in the EMS profession and some not, all who helped me be the person I am. There are many more but not enough space to write about them. I hold a special place in my heart for all of them.

All of the people in EMS whom you are going to read about, work hard and often but miss much of their personal lives, such as little league baseball games and children's plays. And, yet, everyone (ok, almost everyone) understands. This is not a job but a calling.

To those men and women, young and old, black and white, rich and poor, gay and straight, Christian and Jew, I tip my hat and thank you for allowing me to join your ranks.

Our mission has just yet started and we have miles to go before we sleep.

ACKNOWLEDGEMENTS

Tremendous amounts of love and thanks go to my beautiful wife, Barbara, my handsome son, Robert for putting up with my shift work, the overtime that was never ending and the various classes, meetings and other items which took me away from them. I always was thinking of both of you while I worked and wanted to make sure that we had what we needed and that I was there when you needed me to be. I hope I lived up to both of those goals.

I want to thank all of my partners, the good and the bad, for teaching me every day we worked. Lee Godwin, Becky Samples, Bonnie McDonald, Tim Tyus and Mark Elliot. The care we gave our patients will have changed history for so many.

I also want to thank my brother, who is more like a father than a brother. Whether he thinks it or not, he *did* raise me and he did it well. He taught me right from wrong, he listened when I needed him to, never judged, always made me laugh, and among other things, taught me how to sing harmony and, very important to what you are reading now, was instrumental in the editing process. Thanks for the help with editing - although we never got through as much as we would have liked. You have got to upgrade your word processor!!

Everyone has mentors in their life. I am blessed to have a few; Special mentor thanks go out to my brother Walker,

Jay Fitch, Lee Godwin, Bob Hughes, Roland Windham, Pat Browning, George Rice and Donnie Hilliard. They, most likely, would not even know what an impact they have had on my life and so many others. They stand as giants in a world where many "don't want to get involved." Thank you all.

I also want to thank the leaders in the EMS industry who taught me so much. Many are still mentoring to me and others.

Others have left us early but I can't wait until I get to the gate and, should I be allowed to enter (hey, you never know until the gate agent, St. Peter, lets you know if you have a reservation), see these tremendous people again; Ray Graham, Cliff Parker and Jim Algood. All great mentors and close friends. I'll be seeing you one day.

Finally, to the patients, who allowed me into their lives and who's lives I touched - who's hands I held during what certainly was a the scariest moment in your life. Thank you for allowing me the honor of being there for you. You will never know how all of you have changed my life.

1974

He had been getting sleepy. He knew he needed more sleep.

As he drove on Hillsborough Ave., he realized he was only 40 minutes from home. This travel-travel-travel thing was getting old. He thought about his wife and how fantastic she had been during this transition to the new job. His two children, Jenny and Drew, were approaching teen years and we had to get serious about their future. He knew this job would be it – the one which would take him to a higher level.

As he went down the road, his exhaustion got to him. He drifted towards the center of the highway, crossing the double yellow line. He thought about his son's upcoming baseball game. That was the last thing he had in his head when it happened.

. . . .

Brad and Lee sat in their Ambulance at the drive-in, realizing how quiet a night it had been. Two patients, both stable, taken to the ER. Pretty quiet but they both knew what that meant.

"Unit 61," the dispatcher said. There was a sense of urgency in her voice.

"61 is at Dale Mabry and Kennedy," Brad answered.

"We've got a signal 4 out on the causeway. Sounds like a head-on. Rescue is responding with you, possible entrapment," she said.

"10-51," he said. He cranked the engine up and off they went, towards the causeway.

As Brad rode out towards the carnage, with Lee driving, he thought of two things. The first, he wondered, was why hadn't the City, County, or whomever was responsible, put up some barriers for that simple four lane highway. Head-ons were something that happened too many times there, especially late at night. Alcohol almost certainly was involved.

The second thing he thought about was his partner. Lee was a good guy, someone with years of experience, but they had never worked much together. The banter between the two had been friendly and professional. But, this call – it sounded bad and Brad always liked to "know" his partner – his training, his second-guesses, his techniques for trauma. This was the first time they had ever worked together and Brad wanted to get it right. He guessed he would have to learn as they worked.

As he continued to drive with lights and sirens, swerving onto the main road to the Causeway, Lee looked over at his fresh-face partner. Brad, a relatively new EMT, appeared smart, energetic and energized. Lee also knew, sometimes, that a newbie's energy could get in the way of treating the patient, making the right decision. Mistakes out here in the street, were generally very unforgiving, either for the patient, your partner, you –or all three. He would make sure and keep a good eye on him and make sure everyone was on the same plan, the same focus. He'll be fine, Lee thought.

He also started to go through his head about trauma and what he needed to do first. A, B, C Airway, Breathing, Circulation. It was the same for all medical calls. In fact, no one had ever figured out that trauma was an entirely new ballgame. While Airway was important, the only one who was going to fix them was a surgeon. That was, if there was one even in the Hospital at that time of night. Sometimes, they got lucky.

So, Lee knew that time was their enemy. They had to get the patient on the stretcher and hall-butt to the big Hospital. They had all they needed – as long as a surgeon was at the Hospital. He hoped so.

As they approached the scene, it seemed darker than the rest of the highway, although there were no lights to speak of. Then, their headlights hit a part of a car – half of it, it seemed like.

Lee slowed down and both of them stared at what appeared to be one half of a car. It looked like it had been surgically cut in half, with the back portion of it sitting on its rear wheels and on the front metal of the frame, now sitting in the roadway.

No one was inside.

They pulled closer, positioned the Ambulance to protect themselves while out of their Ambulance and both climbed out to find the patients. Even though Brad was somewhat new, the minute he opened the door, he could smell it - fuel, gasoline, and the smell of something burning – not like wood on fire or anything like that. It was like an old engine which was still running but without oil. Metal on metal. He knew that was bad.

Lee jumped from the driver's seat and noted immediately how quiet it was. Sirens were way off in the background, their Fire Department back-up but it would take them several minutes before they arrived. For now, it was just Brad and him.

"Over there," Lee told his partner. Up front, about 200 yards, was the other half of the car they had found. It also was sitting on two front tires, the rear of it sitting on the metal frame.

As Brad approached, he thought he would find someone dead. A surprised look on his and Lees face when they looked in and found no one.

It took Brad a minute to realize, but with his experience, Lee knew – people, most likely, were thrown from the car and out there, either in the brush or maybe in the water. The causeway had the Bay on both sides.

"Hey, look," Brad said to his partner.

Standing over on the side of the road, wavering, was a male in his 30's, clothes torn and hair messed. He was in a suit, his back to us so we couldn't tell what his face looked like.

As they approached him, he turned, and looked at them. A smile came across his face. They could see a cut above his eye and some dirt on his face. "About time you all got here," he said with a smile. "Can you give me a ride home?"

As he approached, the smell of alcohol had faded and Brad didn't notice any near the patient. While that was unusual (50% of the wrecks they went to involved alcohol), it wasn't – at this time of the morning, it *could* be someone who was on the road, late at night – sober.

Brad started immediately to check out the smiling male in the suit, what he certainly thought was the driver of the half-car, asking where he was (he didn't know), what day it was (he thought it was Thursday – wrong) and what City he was in (he told us Atlanta – wrong again). Brad asked if he knew what he had hit (he didn't). The patient told him he "woke up" sitting in the middle of the road with his the front of his half-car sitting behind him. He didn't understand.

Brad asked if he could take his pulse, noticed it was a little fast, felt his skin, noticed it was a little damp (clammy would be the medical term Brad knew), listened to his words, watched his gaze – just like he had been taught.

"Let me get a blood pressure," Brad told the patient. He looked at his partner, "Signal 30?" That meant head injury in code and he was asking his learned partner if he concurred.

Meanwhile, while Lee listened to his partner, watched and concurred, he was also looking down the causeway. Being the senior medical person, he was always looking for something else – the "big picture." Why wasn't there a second car, he wondered. What did they hit? He went back to the Ambulance radio and advised dispatch to start a 2nd unit, afraid of what he would find and not wanting to wait. He also asked the ETA of the cops. They were advised 5 minutes. If they had to search for people, they would need resources on the ground.

While Brad continued treatment, Lee walked over to the front of the half-car and started to walk forward. He knew he might find something he didn't want to find. An entire family, kids, the dog and all, could be in an overturned, mangled car, all dead, or seriously hurt. He had been to enough of them. The fact that their patient didn't seem drunk didn't mean they were out of the woods yet.

He walked about 1,000 yards without finding anything. He went back to the half-car and simply looked out from where the car seemed to come from. Then, seeing a debris field, he walked it to find his other "patient."

Standing tall, unfettered by any vehicle travelling at any speed, was a beautiful palm tree. There was a large gash in it, a front bumper lying to one side and a headlight at its base.

With the exception of the gash, the tree seemed no worse for the wear.

Lee wondered, as he went back to his partner, which way the car had come from. Brad had wrapped a small gash on his patient's wrist and asked Lee to get the stretcher. The Fire Department was arriving now, with Paramedics, and they were doing another evaluation on the same patient. Brad wished that his Paramedic school started sooner.

Fire Rescue – they had Paramedics since 1971. Cool duty, lots of great equipment to help the patient, telemetry radios (Lee really didn't understand all of that but it LOOKED cool) and, of course, IV fluids. Lee didn't know if that would help the patient, but it was cool, none the less.

The fire truck had set up hoses for the gasoline leak in the 2nd half of the car. They had also gotten the long spine board out of the Ambulance and were helping Brad immobilize the patient. That was standard procedure for a possible head injury. Meanwhile, police were on scene, setting up flares (didn't they know there was GASOLINE on the ground? Jeezz!!) and directing traffic around the accident.

As Lee helped the firefighters bring the stretcher over, Brad mentioned that the patient seemed almost manic – and yet was getting sleepier and less coherent (the patient didn't really know where he was when they first found him and now he was repeating questions – a bad sign, according to Lee). His blood pressure hadn't gone down, but the numbers had gotten closer together and his pulse had slowed. It could be two of three of Becks Triade – something Brad had learned in school. When a patients pulse slows down, his blood pressure numbers get closer together and his alertness decreases – those three signs are known as Becks Triade and that is a bad sign of a possible head injury. Man, Brad thought, He sure hope a surgeon is at the Hospital.

With the patient secured to the board and loaded on the stretcher, oxygen applied, they put him in the back. Lee jumped up and said, "Code 3, let's go."

Brad climbed into the front and, with lights flashing, started towards the city Hospital. He knew he had to give his partner a smooth ride, both for the patient and for his field evaluation, which was sure to follow this call. Brad was not surprised when Lee jumped into the patient compartment, even though Lee had driven to the call. He was the senior guy, so he got the choice of driving or riding, whichever and whenever he chose. Since Lee was the more experienced EMT, Brad would drive to the Hospital. Lee had told him that to make sure your emotions didn't translate to how the ambulance is handled when a patient is being transported. Brad made sure to keep his emotions in check. He would give him a baby-skin-smooth ride.

Lee, rechecking vitals, did get a chance to call into the ER and let them know we were coming. He gave them a brief history of what the call was, that the patient had a possible head injury and that we were 25 minutes out. He was hoping they would tell him the surgeon was there.

"10-4", the ER said. "We'll be expecting you."

Lee dreamed of one day having a Hospital with surgeons at the ready, a complete Hospital with everything you needed, X-ray, lab, Neurosurgery, pediatrics, trauma surgeons – the works – all sitting there "on duty" for trauma.

For now, it would have to remain a dream.

"How long?" he yelled up to Brad. Jeez, he thought, it doesn't seem like we're doing any speed.

"5 minutes", Brad said.

Lee was pleased they had made such good time and started to get things ready to move the patient into the ER. The portable oxygen was laid between the patient's legs, a final set of vitals taken, asking the patient again if he knew what day it was, where he was, what had happened. The patient continued to ask Lee if they were going home.

Pulling up to the dock at the ER was a "loading and unloading" process. After all, it was really a dock – at one time, a place where they once unloaded food, sheets and supplies. The good news was when Ambulances backed up to it, they *almost* matched the bottom of the unit floor with the dock. Opening the door from the inside, Lee stepped out as Brad came around.

"Good drive time," he said, complimenting Brad.

Being somewhat pleased at Lee's critique in front of the patient (one who would not remember the entire episode, but that wasn't the point), he unhooked the stretcher and started to roll it out.

"Cannula….**CANNULA!**" Lee shouted. Brad looked up and realized Lee had undone everything – *except* to unhook the oxygen nasal cannula from the unit's oxygen supply and attach it to the portable tank he had taken so much pride in placing on the stretcher.

"Sorry," Lee said sheepishly. Brad would have a great story to tell when the call was over. It's always great when you realize everyone makes mistakes, even the experienced guys.

Lee had a small smile on his face. "I can't believe YOU made me forget that," he said. He was still smiling. "don't let it happen again." Brad didn't know if he was trying to make him feel better or dismissing his error. It did make him feel better to know that everyone makes mistakes.

"Besides", he said with a continued smile. "*We* caught it before we ripped his nose off, so no harm." *We.* As a team, we were both learning but, at that moment, it made Lee a little more vulnerable than I first thought.

They got on each end and manually raised the stretcher to a comfortable position so they could walk it in. As they came through the first doors, Dr. Ramier was waiting for them.

Dr. Ramier, Lee thought. The Podiatrist.

He was a nice-enough doc, Lee thought. He treated the EMTS with respect, as he once was one before he went to medical school.

But seriously, a podiatrist? The patient's feet were fine, it was his head.

"Hi guys, bad night, huh?" the doc asked them.

Lee started to present the patient. "30 year old male, driver in a severe one car accident. Car was split in half. We found him walking on the roadway and he's been asking questions over and over. Not oriented to time and place, no

ETOH (alcohol) on board that we can smell, vitals are stable."

Dr. Ramier listened intently. "Is that all?" he asked.

"Well," Lee said. "His blood pressure. It's stable but the numbers are getting closer together."

Ramier immediately turned to the Nurse walking next to him as they wheeled the stretcher into room 1. "Call Neurosurgery and get someone down here NOW!" he said.

Lee smiled. Ok, so he was a podiatrist, working the midnight shift in the ER, getting a few extra bucks to pay off his medical school loan. At least he knew enough about emergency medicine to call for help when he needed it.

"Thanks," he said to Brad and Lee. "You guys did good."

"We got Dr. Smalls at his home," the Nurse said as she walked back in. "He'll be here in about an hour."

An hour, Lee thought. He could be dead by then.

"An hour?" Ramier asked. "Isn't there anyone closer?"

"No," she replied. "He's the one on call and we only have him."

Ramier looked at us, back at the Nurse, shrugged his shoulders and went to work, starting an IV and ordering blood work and X-rays.

"Is John still here in X-ray?" he asked no one in particular.

"I think so, I'll check" another Nurse said.

As Brad took the stretcher and used equipment back out to the unit, he too wondered when they would fix this crazy system and have a specific Hospital open for serious trauma. Never mind that, he wondered when they would hire REAL emergency room Doctors. The famous "white paper" had been out since 1966, highlighting the deaths from trauma on the highways of the country and what the country needed to fix; 24 hour EMS (Brad had heard of that – he didn't know what that was, but it sure sounded better than an "Ambulance service"); Emergency rooms set up for trauma; Hospitals set up and staffed for trauma; helicopters to quickly move patients to these Hospitals (they were using them in Vietnam – and Maryland – why not here?); and, of course, Paramedic trained folks in the Ambulances. Brad loved being an EMT, but he wanted to learn more, to help more.

Maybe one day, he thought.

Lee came out with the patient chart and asked Brad to read over it.

"Head injury?" Brad asked Lee.

"Yeah, I think so," he answered. There was a discernable pause between the discussions.

"What else?" the more experienced Lee asked his shiny partner.

Brad loved this about Lee. They walked through every call, critiqued it, discussed it, and learned from it. Lee was such a wealth of information and experience. Brad sometimes wished he could just plug himself into Lee's brain and take it all. This "one call at a time" process was slow.

Brad thought for a minute. "Internal injuries?" asking more than stating.

"Internal?" Lee asked. "What signs and symptoms did you have to point to that?"

Brad knew now he was testing him, helping him to learn. He never took offense at any of his questions because he knew, in Lee's heart, he truly wanted to help the EMT learn.

"Well, looking at that car, you've got to assume he's got something wrong inside", Brad said.

"Mechanism of Injury they're calling it," Lee told him and smiled. "I read it in one of the latest articles in Paramedic magazine. Good call."

Brad finished up cleaning up the last of the equipment and getting the unit back into service. Lee checked over the equipment to insure Brad was doing everything he needed to do. As they climbed into the unit, Dr. Ramier came out and shouted to them.

Lee rolled down the window. The Doctor shouted over the engine.

"His spleen is bleeding. We're going to take him to surgery now. Found a surgeon sleeping in the doc room and a gas-passer upstairs doing charts. We're lucky. Thanks for what you did for him."

Lee thought *what I did for him?* "All we did was get him here fast," he told the doc.

"That will probably make all the difference between him living and dying tonight," the doc said and gave us a thumbs up.

As we pulled away, Lee looked at me with those wise eyes.

"Mechanism of injury…." he said – and the Ambulance drove off into the night, awaiting the next call.

ATTITUDE

Dennis was working hard on the shooting patient.

He was young, in fact, the youngest Paramedic, at the time, in the entire State. 18 years old and here he was, hovering over a 20-something male with a gunshot wound to the chest.

"Pretty cool shooting, eh?" he asked to no one in particular.

The patient looked up at him, pretty ticked at his description of his calamity.

Dennis, in his excitement, had forgotten the patent was still awake.

. . . .

"They are all douchbags," Ken said. He was loading a patient, a female found in the street, unconscious. The smell of stale wine emanated from her, a week's worth of dirt caked on her face.

Clearly, she had seen better days.

So had her 8 year old son, who had been standing next to her when the word "douchbag" rolled off of Ken's tongue, talking about his mother.

. . . .

The ER Doctor stood at the entrance to the room as the Paramedic rolled another psychiatric patient into his ER.

"Why do you keep bringing these patients to me?" he asked. "Don't you understand this is an *emergency* room? I don't want to treat your trash today or ever. Take it on over to County."

The medic, tears in his eyes, leaned down to his father and whispered, "Don't worry Dad. He's always like that."

. . . .

Each of these real situations is rolling through my mind as I walk through our local airport, on the way to catch a flight to Denver.

They are doing a major overhaul and, as a result, the closest entrance to my airline desk is closed. As I walk further up to the new temporary entrance, I realize I'll have to walk back down the same length, past all of the other airlines, to get to mine. As inconvenient as it is, it will tell me a story about life and attitude that I think I already knew, but certainly showed itself in what I observed.

As I turn into the main building I start walking by various "other" airlines. I notice several things. Most have professionals waiting for their next customer. Then, I walk up to a popular discount airline and I notice something different.

People there are laughing, smiling, actually looking like they are enjoying being there and doing what they are doing. They look like a team, a group of individuals with the same mission, that of making the customer happy.

They have happy faces, a happy looking counter, party favors around them – it's obvious that they are "hunting" for customers, telling them with only a visual cue that *they* are the airline to fly. Fun. Satisfied. Happy.

I walk past them to my airline. I like them, don't get me wrong. They are also happy, smiling, fun. They are a little put back, not as "happy" as the previous discount airline, but obviously knowing that the desk before them, of which all of their customers much temporarily travel by, looks *happier*.

Then, there are the others. Pan-faced, leaning against something, looking as if they would rather be anywhere but there. No music, no smiling faces, no party favors. Now, don't get me wrong, once customer approaches, they perk up – as if on cue – and give a great greeting.

Like a machine. Like it's something they *have to do*.

. . . .

Attitudes, especially in EMS, are pretty standard. For the most part, a majority of EMS practitioners really want to be there. It is not a job for them but a calling. They have acknowledged, to themselves, that they are not going to get rich doing what they are doing. Nor are they going to get famous. They do this work because it must be done and must be done by someone who cares for those in need, those rich and poor, of all races and sexes and lifestyles. They have no judgments on the lives of others because, if they are true caregivers and true to themselves, they know that "there but for the grace of God go I."

In this business, attitude is *everything*. Those of us who are serious about patient care realize that our sole purpose in our mission is to serve others. We are a servant to the sick and injured and, even when they are a little salty in their language and attitude, our attitude must remain as a servant to them – to all.

There are those, however, who did *not* get into this position to care for anyone, unless it was a call that, in their opinion, *really needed us*. That means a shooting, car crash (not a neck pain but serious trauma), knifing, explosion or mass casualty (with lots of *cool* trauma).

These folks are not into it to *care* for patients and, certainly, aren't servants. In fact, they are insulted that anyone would even refer to them in that way. They think a servant is subordinate to them and, in their mind, does not ring the true, *heroic* (read - *god-like*) sense of what they think their mission is.

We have these folks in all walks of life. We look at them at work and wonder what they are doing there. *If they hate it so much, why do they stay?*

An interesting question.

These folks also have a tendency to stay somewhere because, simply, *it's easier.* They don't want to take any risks (less they mess it up and get blamed) or try anything that may be new to them, hence it makes it look as if they didn't know *everything about everything.* To them, they are there to drive fast, turn on the red lights and be the hero at the scene, the big uniformed king to will save a life (*if,* in their opinion, a life is worth saving).

These folks bitch about everything from the elected officials, to the Director, to their Supervisors (*especially about the leadership)* to their own co-workers. They gravitate to like-kind negative-Nellie's who will confirm their depressing thoughts.

Eventually, you see them in their own circle of two or three life-haters, and for the most part, no one else can stand to be around them anymore.

I have a theory, which you can probably tell, is not that positive.

For years, we recruited EMTs by telling them they should get the training and come to work for us *to save a life.* That was a little disingenuous.

We now know that you come to work to *care for others*. In the 20-30 years you work in this profession, there *may* be a time that you actually get to save a life.

However, *being a servant to others* is the meat and potatoes of what we do.

The other, saving a life, is the gravy.

There are lots of other great things about this profession. You learn a great deal about the human body and how it works (or sometimes doesn't). You learn a great deal of technology to help them in their hour of need and gain a pile of common sense ideas on how to handle an emergency.

We do *not* make a million dollars and, in fact, many of us barely make ends meet. Some of that is self-driven (I want the toys) and, for others, it is simply how EMS currently is.

Even with all of that, a good attitude is absolutely something you have to have, up front, on deck, all of the time.

So, let me give you an example, based upon six different people I have worked with, or led, in four different organizations.

As I begin, you should note that throughout this book, I commonly refer to people who work with me as *co-*

workers. That's because I dislike the word *employee*. It sounds – well, just wrong.

However, for those we are going to talk about for a minute, they are employees and you'll see why at the end.

Employee #1 is a 40 something veteran who went so far as to get his intermediate EMT. Throughout his career, he has not taken very good care of himself, has become overweight and tired of what he does.

"When you see those mullet flopping around," he would start when talking about an epileptic. "It's the funniest thing you've ever seen." His smile shows his smirk for those suffering from the disease.

When everyone else's morale is up, he is the most miserable. When everyone is down, he is the happiest.

He had a tragedy in his life involving a family member, everyone will tell you, and he has never been the same. He is so negative; no one will eat with him or even be near him (except fellow negatives).

The sad thing is, this man is an excellent care-giver. I have watched him taking care of people who he would no more give the time of day than the man in the moon. He smiles, cares, serves.

Why is this guy such a problem? Because most people, including the patient, can see the fakeness in his care. He's going through the motions, taking care of people because –

well, that's what is on the script. No compassion. No caring, Just rote action.

Why he doesn't quit and go do something he likes I will never know. But, he never realized how miserable he was making everyone else.

Employee # 2 had worked for the service for a few years and quit because he didn't like what he was doing. He felt the management staff were idiots and he could no longer stand the craziness. That management staff, by the way, is all the way from his immediate Supervisors through and up to the elected officials.

After a few years of working as his own boss (self-employment is somewhat of a *bitch* since your one and only employee you have to really satisfy is yourself, a hard thing to do when you loath your life), he asked to return to EMS. This is after a complete change of leadership.

However, nothing had changed for this employee. He hated many Supervisors he worked with, hated all of the command staff and didn't think much about his patients.

Many who had been in the service for 30+ years said he had been like that when he had worked for us before and were, quite frankly, surprised when we had hired him back.

But, there he was, hating everything about what he did and, particularly, who he worked with and for.

Eventually, he would go out on a disability, unable to deal with the *stress* of the job (or of his bad attitude).

Most of us agreed he drove himself to that *life* and never left.

Employee # 3 had been promoted to a Supervisor position and held a high standard for everyone under her leadership – except herself.

She was constantly late for her shift and always insured that she had the *inside track* to what was happening. At one point, she was able to get the ear of a senior management staff, above command staff, for requests and rumor control (or uncontrol). Once, in front of her direct Supervisor, she spoke on the phone to another co-worker, spreading a rumor about someone who worked with them.

She ruled with an emotional fist, making sure that those who she liked ended up *being taken care of* and those she did not, not.

She was, what we called, the *emotional whirlwind.*

Eventually, those who were her friends drew away from her, many telling us later that they simply couldn't take all of her drama. After all, everyone had enough drama in watching those patients they cared for without making it up in-house.

The # 4 employee was probably one of my biggest disappointments. He came to us as an EMT, we sent him to

Paramedic school and, upon exiting, he didn't have much faith in his own ability to write good reports. Through much hard work with many co-workers, he did well. He ended up on a high professional position, but eventually came back to Paramedic medicine.

So, what's wrong with this attitude? Well, let's just say that his high professional position was actually a Physician. Yes, this employee went through and graduated from medical school, but decided not to complete his residency. Instead he returned to EMS.

And, with it, a *Doctors personality* (I apologize to all of those great Doctors who *don't* think they are perfect) which could not admit or even fathom that he may have made a mistake.

Once, when a question (not even a definite issue, just a question) regarding the care of a patient came from our Medical Director (himself a Doctor), this employee screamed so that everyone could hear, that he was being *tried* by the system.

While he pointed out to the Medical Director that he had *never* had a report returned for a documentation issue, he failed to note that he took 35% longer to complete those reports than the earliest rookie.

So, in conclusion, what do all of these employees have in common? A failure to have a positive attitude, about their work, about their team and about their patients. They think by smiling at them, while laughing behind their backs (I was talking about their co-workers, not their patients), that makes it ok.

The reasons for these attitudes are as numerous as the causes. The one common view, however, across the spectrum, is that they are unhappy with their own lives, how they turned out, how happy everyone else seems with their life and how unfair everything is.

They are life-sucking, energy draining bags of annoying hell. And, for their own misgivings, everyone around them must suffer.

As I walk back from my airline counter past the discount airline, they are still there, smiling, cracking jokes, saying hello to everyone who passes. Caring, Happy, Customer oriented.

Attitude is everything in this business, more than the medicine you do, bigger than the Ambulance you drive. It will send you to heights you can only imagine or cause you to crash into a career that you will hate with a vengeance.

And, after all, why would you want to stay there?

DOUGHNUT SALAD

Of the many houses we go into on a regular basis, there is nothing quite like going into a house at the dead of night, filled with people who don't speak your language.

In Tampa, where my professional career started, there were many Cuban families and many didn't know how to speak English. This has always been a challenge for us trying to get medical information on someone who may be dying. The days of EMTs and Paramedics taking another language, or even knowing one when they came into the business, was rare. Translation, in many instances, was not an option.

Yes, I know I should have paid more attention in Spanish class in High School. Only years later when I took a trip to Guatemala did I discover that *conversational Spanish* was not taught – instead, nouns and verbs and just enough to get you in trouble if you tried to use it.

Yes, we could have taken a class or two in Spanish after we became certified, but it was all we could do to learn the medical side of Paramedicine. Things changed every day and new drugs were being issued and procedures initiated. Spanish was an option but it was not at the top of the list.

I cannot count the amount of calls we were dispatched on in which I never found out what the real issue was. I know that sounds crazy, but getting them to the Emergency

Room (ER), in those instances, was quicker than trying to find someone who could translate.

It wasn't only Cuban issues. We had our fair share of Chinese, Russian and Mexican (no, that's not the same as Cuban, believe me). Today, we have an 800 number to call to get an instant translator. In those days, it was poking and prodding and hoping someone in the house knew English as their 2nd language.

I believe the one night that sits in my mind was when my partner, Tim, and I went to the house on another planet and attempted to treat someone who, as their second language, did not have command of said language.

Combine that with my partner who was previous in stage 3 REM sleep (deep, DEEP sleep for you non-REM folks) and you have two people learning their own language (and possibly someone else's). The interpretation is what caught us.

Being in that deep of a sleep at work was pretty unusual for a Paramedic because most of us slept with one eye open during the shift. Even though there are beds in the station, the idea that you get a "good night's sleep" is pretty much unheard of. With all of the bells, alarms, radios, telephones et al ringing, buzzing and ding-a-linging all night, you were lucky if you got 20 minutes sleep. You also had that dreaded fear that you would sleep through a call and that generally kept you at a "doze" mode of sleep.

I have to stop for a minute and mention one slight divergence from that scenario. In the stations where we shared quarters with the Fire Department, those guys had NO PROBLEM sleeping at night. How do I know that, you say? Well, two areas tell me that was so.

First, the volume and amount of snoring that went on from the fire side of the bunk room told me that a bomb couldn't wake most of the guys who rode the big red truck.

The second, however, was more telling.

Every bunk room had speakers in which the fire radio would announce when a fire was occurring. EMS, on the other hand, had small portable radios and pagers for our calls.

The fire radio speakers are set at the volume of STUN (or Cardiac as some of us say), loud enough to cause deafness, or chest pain, when they went off.

And, even at that volume, at that ear splitting level, I was amazed at the amount of firefighters who never woke up for the call. Of course, the others would yell and scream (hence why Paramedics in fire stations rarely got six straight hours of sleep) but they wouldn't budge. After two minutes, the remainder of the guys would take off on the truck, leaving the unfortunate firefighter to get the wrath *from* god (or the Chief as he is lovingly called) when it was realized that said firefighter was not on scene.

Although my partner was not a firefighter, nor did he get any better sleep than most of us, on that particular night, Tim was, in fact, VERY asleep – as I said, stage 4 REM sleep. That is a fancy way of saying that Tim had no idea where he was, who he was with, what he was doing or what planet he was on.

On a good way to enter into an emergent situation, but it is what it is.

We worked on 410, which had a large commercial area, but had quite a few suburban areas, in the outskirts of our district. We could tell what area we were going to by which way we turned out of the station.

We were dispatched around 2 AM to a house that had those familiar burglar bars on every window, however, except for that, it looked pretty ordinary. I was the lead medic (Tim and I swapped every other call) and, as we pulled up to the yard, noted the fire engine already on scene. I grabbed my equipment and started towards the front door.

The process, normally, is that you see fire folks with your patient and you always assume that your partner is right behind you, bringing in the remainder of what may be needed.

The fire captain shrugged his shoulders. "I don't know," he said. "They don't speak English."

The male appeared to be in distress of some sort. I leaned down to hand calmly talked to him.

"Can you tell me what the problem is this morning?" He looked at me and moaned, rapidly breathing the oxygen the fire folks had started.

"He has been having chest pain for a couple of hours," the woman with him said. She had a very heavy Cuban accent but appeared to understand what I was asking.

The fire guys looked at me, surprised as they hadn't talked to her, but everyone appeared a little less panicked since we had someone who understood our language. They moved aside so I could get in and talk to her.

"Are you his wife?" I asked. She said "Si" and it seemed everything was getting better, communications-wise.

"Ask him where his pain is – point to it with his finger," I told her. She did and he pointed to just over his stomach. Chest pain is commonly used when the pain actually is somewhere south of that. Everyone saw where he was pointing and, although we weren't out of the forest yet, we calmed a bit more. Things seemed to be going well.

"Do you take any medications we need to know about?" I asked. This was a common question asked of all Patients. He nodded no. The wife confirmed he didn't.

"So, did the pain wake him up?" I asked his wife. "What happened after he told you about the pain?"

"Well," she said a matter of fact. "I gave him the nitroglycerin."

I stared at her.

"So, he takes nitro?" I asked, a little irritated but still engaged in finding what the problem was.

"Yes, he takes nitro," she said, a little irritated.

Ok, I thought. Maybe the wife and he didn't understand that was a medication. Whatever.

"What happened after that?" I asked.

"Well," the wife continued. "That didn't help so I gave him some donasol." It seemed like she slurred the name of what she had given him and none of us knew what that was. The Cuban accent didn't help. I didn't understand what donasol was and was going to ask when my partner, Tim, suddenly appeared from the outside, coming through the door and appearing like someone who had just been slapped by their girlfriend.

Remember, I had woken him up at 2 AM in stage 4 REM sleep. I wasn't sure he was awake yet. By his statement, I realized he was not.

"*DOUGHNUT SALAD?*" he asked, very loudly. "What the hell does that mean, you gave him a doughnut salad?"

Just by itself, it made no sense to anyone standing around the patient, but the line was so funny, all of us started to laugh.

That didn't sit well with the wife.

"No," the wife said, sounding rather flustered. "Donasol." She said it again and I couldn't understand.

"Do you mean Donatol?" I queried.

"Yes, Donatol" she said, exhausted at trying to make us understand what she was saying.

He takes Donatol?" I asked, also exhausted at the entire issue of questions. She shook her head.

OK, I thought. He takes two medicines and she clearly said he was not taking any medication. I felt a tap on my shoulder. It was Tim, still looking sleepy.

Everyone in the room realized that I was somewhat ticked.

"Is there any other medication he takes that we need to know about?" I asked one more time.

Before the wife could answer (she was already shaking her head no and I knew that was no longer a valid answer), I felt Tim tapping me on the shoulder. Still looking like a stunned half-asleep puppy, he looked straight at me. It looked like his eyes were open but no one was at the controls.

"You're asking it wrong," he said, matter of fact. He looked at the wife.

"Is there any other medication that he *doesn't* take that we **don't** need to know about?"

The question made no sense to me but the wife's face opened up as if communication had been made.

"YES," she announced. "There's a whole table full of medicine he doesn't take that you don't need to know about."

Tim looked at me and smiled. "I'll get the stretcher."

While we prepared the patient for transport, I walked out to the dining room table and saw a plethora of pill bottles, many of the same medication. It took about 5 minutes to write down the names and dosages but it appeared that most of them were for a stomach issue.

The patient was loaded on the stretcher and placed in the back of the Ambulance.

"Do you know where we are going?" I asked, seeing if the wife had told us a facility of preference.

"Well, unless you want to take him back to the station, I suggest we go to the Hospital," Tim said without a smile on his face. I still don't think he was awake yet.

"You do know which one, right?" I asked one more time, smiling because the line was so funny but exhausted at repeating questions two and three times.

"Centro Auspurian Hospital," he said.

Of course.

The local Cuban-owned, membership-only Hospital, was a small community Hospital that had a one bed ER and a Cuban Physician who lived on site for members who came to be admitted.

We transported the patient, with his translator in the back, to the Hospital without incident.

However, ever since that call, when Tim or I ask a waitress to bring us a *doughnut salad*, we both fall on the floor laughing.

They don't get it.

It's a Paramedic thing.

1969

It started as an ache.

As Mr. Jerrystone sat down to read the paper, he noted the pain – not really pain, sort of discomfort – right under the base of his breast bone.

His wife saw his face and asked him, "John, are you ok?"

"Oh yeah," he said. "Just some gas."

Within the next 20 minutes, she noticed he had started to sweat and turn a pale kind of – well, she couldn't put her finger on it, but it seemed he was actually turning grey.

Knowing he was in trouble, she got up and walked over to the phone book and opened it to the yellow pages.

"Ambulance, Ambulance…..now, where is it?" she asked. The Ambulance in town was run by the local Funeral Home – they had gotten magnets from them during the town fair but, at that moment, she couldn't find it on the refrigerator.

She finally found Ralphs Funeral Home and called the number. It seemed like it rang a long time.

"Ralphs Funeral Home, can I help you?" the calm voice answered.

"Yes, this is Maggy Jerrystone over on 5th place and I think my husband is having a heart attack." She thought for a moment – I don't know why I said that, I don't know a thing about what I'm talking about – but he looks so *sick*.

She told the man on the phone the address and he conveyed that they would be right over.

"Do you all carry oxygen?" she asked. She didn't know why she asked that either, but thought it would be good to have if they did.

"Yes mam', oxygen equipped and radio dispatched," the man said, as if he was making a commercial.

"Thank you and please hurry" she told the man.

Jack Harris had just started his shift at the Funeral Home. He was wearing his new suit especially for the large funeral that they had scheduled for later in the day. He looked sharp.

He had barely been there 20 minutes when the telephone call came in for an Ambulance run.

Immediately, he wondered if the hearse had anyone in it. Normally, the staff always left it empty but there were occasions when a "customer" had come in early in the morning and hadn't been removed yet. He hoped that wasn't the case, since he was the only one there.

He hurried to get the keys and went out to set the hearse up. Opening the rear door, he was pleased to note that there wasn't anyone using it – and climbed in to pull the dark curtains back behind the posts of the vehicle. He then exited and went to get the stretcher.

He was happy that they had just bought a new "kicker" stretcher that one person could use. There were so many times they only had one person in the hearse – I mean Ambulance – and newer stretcher seemed easier to use. He loaded it in the Ambulance, placed the red light on the top and took off for the address.

On the way, he realized he had forgotten to lock the door but figured other staff would be in by 9 AM that morning – he had forgotten to leave a note of where he was going and no one was there to answer the radio. Oh well – they'll figure it out.

He arrived to find what looked like the wife, waiving him down frantically.

"He's in there and he looks bad," he yelled.

He grabbed the stretcher out of the back of the hearse, loaded the first aid kit on the cot, and steered them into the house. Luckily, there were no stairs to climb. He hated to ask a relative to help him get the bed into the house.

Upon entering, he realized this was serious. Across the room sat Jerry, gray and cold, sweaty and with labored breathing. He was in serious trouble.

"How you doing, partner?" he asked, as upbeat as he could while not showing how scared *he* was.

"Trouble.....breathing....pressure..." was all he could get out.

Jack pulled out the plastic oxygen mask and hooked it up to the regular.

.....*what did they say – heart attack, as much oxygen as you could give him.....when he's blue, give him the works*.....

He noted that although John was grey, that was closer to blue than normal so he put the oxygen at 20 liters. Air rushed out into the mask and onto John's face.

"Breath that oxygen – it will help you," he said to the man who was dying.

He asked the patient to get up and swing around to the stretcher, which he had now placed at floor level. *Gosh, I wish the stretcher had more than two positions – all the way up or all the way down*....and had John sit on the stretcher. He tried to lay him down but he couldn't breathe. He sat the back up and that helped.

Now, although he could maneuver the stretcher out to the Ambulance, he realized he couldn't lift it on his own. He couldn't ask the wife – she was too small and really scared.

He got the stretcher to the back of the unit and walked around to the front. He hit the siren once, loud and came back to the patient.

"Don't worry," he said. "I'm just getting some help."

Within 2-3 minutes, several men came out of the neighborhood houses, looking to see what was happening.

"Hey, guys, give me a hand, could ya?" he asked.

Without question, three men came over and helped lift the stretcher to the load position.

From there, he could shove it towards the rear, causing the legs to collapse towards him and the stretcher to lower itself about 3 inches to the floor of the floor of the unit. The legs folded up and he was able to load the stretcher into the back.

Climbed in and adjusted the mask again. "Stay calm and let the oxygen help you" he told John. He looked into the patient's eyes and realized how much in trouble he really was.

"I'm going to go up front and drive," and, with that, he climbed out and closed the door. He told the wife to follow, but not too close.

"We don't want another patient, now do we?" he calmly said, smiling and trying to give a piece of calmness to what he knew was a very scary situation.

He started to the Hospital, getting out onto the main highway and gaining speed. The 454 engine in the hearse could really get up some speed and pretty soon they were pegging 80 MPH.

During the ride, continued to yell into the back, "How's that oxygen doing for you" – and it really didn't matter how it *was* doing for him, as long as he was still answering. Most of the time you couldn't hear what the patients were saying, especially with the oxygen mask on. It wasn't really important, though, because your job was to get him to the Hospital quickly. They could really *do something* if you could just get the patient there.

Jack wheeled into the emergency room, siren blaring – shutting it off as soon as he entered the Hospital parking lot, adhering to the Nurse's request that noise be kept to a minimum near the Hospital. The last siren noise would at least alert the ER.

Pulling up to the door, one Nurse had come out and he gave her the "bad sign" that he had a critical patient. She ran back in to get an orderly and reappeared with a large man in a white tunic.

Even before Jack could get to the rear door, the orderly had opened it and started to pull the stretcher out.

"Stop", Jack said. He didn't know this orderly and was afraid he wouldn't know how to work the under carriage. It wouldn't be the first time someone who was only trying to help threw the patient and stretcher down onto the driveway.

Jack pulled the wheels out and leveled the stretcher. Both men steered it into the Emergency room to the one of two beds for critical patients.

"What have you got?" the Nurse asked. She had the telephone in her hand to give the doc a call. He was, most likely, asleep or in the Doctor's lounge.

"Heart attack," Jack shouted. It seems strange that in our training, they specifically told us that we *couldn't* diagnose. It was against the law. We would be practicing medicine. We would be hung.....

The Nurse finished dialing and spoke into the phone. She hung up and came into the treatment room.

"15 liters of oxygen? That's way too much," she said. She pulled out a nasal cannula and placed it on the oxygen outlet, dialing it at 4 liters per minute. She stuck the nose prongs into the patient's face and slipped the holder over his ears.

"You EMT's," she said, shaking her head. A moment later, the Doctor entered.

He seemed like a good guy, looking like he had been woken up from a good sleep, looking over the patient and then to the Nurse.

"Chest Pain?" he asked.

"Yes, Doctor," the Nurse said. "I put him on 4 Liters of oxygen." No mention of what Jack had done, but what the heck.

Jack walked out with the stretcher and went to the back of the Hearse....er, Ambulance. He took some fresh linen from the ER and made up the stretcher, put it back into the Ambulance, grabbed his pad and went back into the treatment room.

When Jack got there, there was another Nurse who had come down from ICU. They were hanging IV's, getting EKGs and making notes. Jack didn't know what MS was (I later found out it was Morphine) but they were giving him quite a bit to ease the pain.

Jack went back out to the waiting room where the wife stood by herself, looking like her best friend had just left here. It might actually happen tonight.

"Mam'," he stated.

"How is he?" she lunged at me.

"The Doctors are working on him now", Jack replied. Rule # 1 was never to tell the family what was *really* going on – that the ER was working hard at something but they weren't equipped or educated to know what to do next either.

Jack got some information from the wife, name, address, date of birth, and then came the most uncomfortable part of his job.

"Mam', you know that Ralphs Funeral Home does this as a service to the community without government money," he stated. "The bill for the Ambulance is $25.00 and $5.00 for the oxygen," She started to reach into her purse.

"However," he said. "I am authorized to make the Ambulance call free of charge to your husband, provided you sign here."

It was a statement that, when the time arrived, she would call us to make arrangements for her husband.

She read it without even flinching and signed. Jack smiled, said thank you and gave her hopes that he would pull through.

Ghoulish, you say? Maybe - but it was the only system out there. The local government didn't have the money and the State and Federal governments didn't think it was their job to fund it. So, the only people who could do Ambulance services were the volunteer rescue squads and Funeral Homes. It was one of their business models. It served the public in a way no one else could and ensured business could be steered towards your Funeral Home in the future.

Jack walked out just as the Doctor exited the rear of the ER.

"Man, that's a bad one," he told Jack. "Worse I've seen who managed to stay alive to the ER."

"What chances does he have?" Jack asked.

"Pretty good if I can get a Cardiologist in here," he said. "After all, I'm a podiatrist just working some extra hours in the ER."

Jack got into the Ambulance and pulled out to return to the Funeral Home.

And, so it was in 1969.

NOBODY MESSES WITH MY SISTERS

The house was silent.

Lying in a pile of freshly folded clothes now tangled and blood-soaked on the ground of the main hallway, a man's body was spread as far as the walls of the hallway would allow a single cluster of buckshot in the center of his back. The color of his shirt, like the color of the newly washed clothes piled under him, appeared to darken more red with each passing minute.

In a small bedroom right off of where the dead man lay, two little girls sleep peacefully in their beds, oblivious to the action that had just taken place in the small, wooden house.

Up near the front of the house, sitting on a couch, was a nine year old, holding the instrument of death, the shotgun his grandfather had left him just before he died.

"This is for you, grandson," his grandfather had told him one night. "This is only to be used to protect your family."

And now, the boy sat, after making the call to the police. The air was heavy with the smell of gun powder and sweat. He heard the sirens in the background, wondering what would happen to him. Would he be arrested? Is the man dead?

The sirens got closer.

At first, he glanced towards the front of the house and saw the slit screen on the front door. Then, he glanced back towards the body and saw that the blood had now spread to all of the clean clothes under him.

He grimaced. His Mom was sure going to be mad about that.

....

Our shift started like any other. Being on night shift, things were already picking up in the city and checking off our supplies was a work in progress. The changeover at night was difficult and always an action in motion.

The crew change took place something like this; your assigned unit came in, fresh from the field and the day shift, and parked at the gas pump. While the driver got out and started to fuel it up, the new crew would start throwing their personal stuff inside the cab, throwing out the old from the crew before. The Crew Chief from the day shift left and went to supply immediately to get the resupply order completed. The fresh crew would either get a report of the mechanical items (from the driver) or start checking the larger items (oxygen level, suction working, stretcher inside – ok, that last one was a bit of a joke, but you *never knew* what you would or would not find when you opened the doors).

If it sounds a little rough – throwing the other crews things out onto the sidewalk – Well, we didn't exactly "throw" the stuff, but we did have to get it all out before the unit caught another call. Nothing worse than to see the new crew drive off, red lights blaring, and realize that your wallet (or worse yet – your car keys) were still in the Ambulance.

Then, there were those nights when it was quiet. There weren't many of them, but when they happened, it was crazy as well. The difference is that the units were lined up behind each other, waiting to use the one fuel pump we had at the time. No one could go home until the unit was refueled and cleaned. Overtime was at a premium and the company certainly didn't want you spending that on anything other than a money making endeavor (picking up a patient who would be paying for the transport). Cleaning and fueling, in management's opinion, should be done "on your time."

Luckily for us, the federal government disagreed.

Anyhow, this particular night appeared to be relatively quiet and our unit had been the first one in and, as a result, the first one out. The night grinded on and we were doing our thing. Dispatch had sent us to a few calls, nothing outrageous or super hard. The drone of the radio got quieter around 1 AM.

My partner, John, and I had not worked a great deal together. He was really a cool guy, much older than most of us, but wise with years. He had been a dispatcher for the

State Police and decided he wanted to help people. He was a good partner to have, someone who made sure you were never in danger and that the patient always got taken care of.

The greatest thing about John was his ability to tell stories. It would seem that the strangest, most exciting, most gut-wrenching calls were all his and the way he could tell the story had you sitting on the edge of your seat. You couldn't believe one guy could have this much excitement during his tour of duty.

This tour was to be no different for John.

Around 3 AM, we had been parked downtown, covering the zone, when the radio blared of a shooting. They assigned it to us and we booked towards that like the adrenalin junkies that we were. "A shooting", we both thought. Now, THERE was a call you could do something on. Save a life. Stop the bleeding. Who knows, the TV station might even be there and you could end up on the morning news.

Hey, look – I never said we all didn't have egos!

In those days, we did not wait for the cops to arrive before we went into a potentially dangerous scene. Now, as I read what I just wrote, I am thinking, "What in the world were we doing? However, it was a different time and scene safety was not on the top of the list for most agencies.

It was, however, for the crews. As we drove emergency to the scene, the usual check lists went through our minds. Check for scene safety, find the cops, make sure no one was still shooting, find the cops, find the cops…..

It was a plain, small, regular type of house. It had a screen porch on it. It looked like any other house on the street. I remember pulling up. Police cars were everywhere but none stood outside. Unusual, I thought. I grabbed the jump kit, a small first aid kit with whatever we would need to stabilize the patient prior to getting them to the unit. John grabbed the oxygen and we entered.

As we walked through the porch door, there were cops looking at a cut screen and a fingerprint technician brushing dust all over the front of the door. Inside, there was the second entrance into the main house. When you opened that door, you realized that the hallway you were entering went all the way to the back of the house. There was the living room, which was to our immediate right and two doorways off of the hallway near the back. One to the left and one almost at the rear.

As we passed the living room, there were several Officers there, surrounding what appeared to be a small child. He looked around nine years old. He was sitting on the only couch in the room. We started to go towards the boy, assuming he was the one shot, when the cop who was looking at us held his hand out as if to block our access to him.

He motioned for us to continue towards the back of the house.

As we continued down the hallway, lit with one small light bulb and many hand held police flashlights, we found our victim. A short, adult male, face down in the center of the intersection of the hallway and the doorway to the left, laying on what appeared to be freshly folded clothes. They were soaked in what appeared to be the victim's blood.

For a moment, we went into auto-mode.

"Check for a pulse," John told me and we both kneeled down near the patient's head.

Trying to keep the crime scene untouched while treating a patient can be challenging. In this case, it wasn't that hard. Although we were both preparing to do a primary patient check (airway, circulation (pulse), respiration), we could both tell without touching him that he was dead. The large blood stain under him was soaking the clothes and the fact that, when we rolled him a piece of his chest was missing, gave us hints that he was no longer alive.

After checking for a pulse, breathing and seeing that the wound was momentous, he rolled him back into the position found and looked up at the cops.

"Signal 7", I confirmed, using the radio code for DOA. It was so strange – No matter who I worked with, we never used plain language when we spoke to each other. It was like a secret language we had. WE knew what we were saying but we thought no one else did.

We then saw the shot gun shell out in front of the man, looking lonely and used. I looked further up from that and that's when I saw them.

In one of the two rooms that came off of the hallway, there were two little girls, sleeping in twin beds. They looked so peaceful and quiet. With the noise and confusion in the house due to what had occurred, the view of that serene scene in the one room of the house caused the entire scene to be somewhat skewed.

Outside, in the main hallway, and in the living room, radios on police Officers hips yelled and made noise, People stepped around and over this dead body in the doorway. The crime lab was there, now taking flash pictures.

Eight feet away, innocence slept.

We stepped back from the body, noting for the Detective who was now hovering over me, where I specifically touched the body and then backed out into the front room. I looked back over and noticed that the small boy hadn't moved from the place we had seen him when we entered. Now, the huddle of Officers around the boy had dispersed. He hadn't looked at us, or at the cop who remained, or it appeared, anyone else. He seemed small, quiet, somehow at peace – but not. Like the little girls in the other room – but not.

Now, we started to think. Was this his Dad? Had someone come in and killed his father in front of the boy? Is it his baby-sitter, confronting a home invader and protecting the children?

I handed the jump kit to John and started towards the boy. As I approached, the lone police Officer moved aside as if he knew my intent.

"Are you OK?" I asked.

His name was Tyson. He looked up at me and simply said, "Yeah."

I started to do a patient assessment, as we would anyone at a scene who might be hurt. As I grabbed for his pulse, he pulled his arm back.

"Hey," he said. "I said I'm ok."

"Sorry," I muttered. I had broken one of my primary rules – never touch a patient until you tell them what you are going to do. "I just wanted to make sure you weren't hurt."

"What happened?" I gulped, finally realizing I had to get some kind of story.

"He didn't even blink. "I shot that man", he said.

To say that statement set me back is an understatement.

A nearby Officer pulled me aside.

"That's the Uphill delivery guy", he said, as if I was supposed to know what that meant. The Uphill Delivery Service was a national company that delivered packages.

The first thing to my mind; what was he doing here at 3 AM delivering a package?

My confusion showed in my face and triggered the cop that I was lost as to what this entire scene was.

"He delivered a package today and made some moves on the mom", he continued. "She told him to get lost and I guess he came back after hours."

Now, I was both shocked and mad. I also realized why the screen door had been cut.

The Officer continued. "He evidently was starting to sneak into that room (he pointed towards the room with the two little girls) and started towards there. I don't know why. Maybe he thought Mom would be there."

"That's when he shot him", he said and pointed to the Nine year old.

"Where's the mom?" I asked.

"She works nights," he said matter of fact. "Tyson is the man of the house when she is gone."

I tried to fathom being Nine years old and being the man of the house." I went to when I was nine and realized I didn't know the floor from the ceiling and certainly didn't know how to hold a shotgun, no less shoot one.

I walked back over to the couch Tyson hadn't moved from. He had his knees pulled up and tucked under his chin.

"Hey, Tyson," I asked. "Tell me what happened."

Again, he never blinked. He turned his head towards me. "I heard him jiggling the door. Then I heard him cut the screen. I knew who it was. He looked like a bad guy when he was here earlier. I snuck into the closet where the shotgun was and waited. I saw him enter the hallway and start towards my sisters. I yelled, "Hey!" and he turned so I could get a good look at him. I shot at him and he fell."

As I heard the words coming out of this boy's mouth, I realized that although he was physically only nine, he sounded and acted much older than his years.

"Mom's going to be mad," he said as an afterthought. "She just washed those clothes."

Again, I stared in awe.

Several minutes went by without anyone saying much of anything. Finally, the boy broke the uncomfortable silence.

"Is he dead?" he asked.

"Yes, Tyson, he's dead," I told him.

Another shorter silence.

"Good," he answered.

The answer wasn't angry, nor was it the kind of "final word" you think you would hear. Instead, it was sort of thinking *out loud* comment.

Then, he looked at me with his little boy eyes and his stern and somewhat wise looking face and, without blinking an eye, gave me a piece of information that, even though the Officers had a theory of what had occurred, they had yet to get a statement from the boy.

"He was walking into my sister's room. He was gonna mess with my sisters," he said.

One more silence. Then, as sternly as one would make an absolute statement. He looked straight at me without anger and without remorse.

"Nobody's gonna' mess with my sisters,"

We stayed around for a few minutes until the Mom arrived from work. The car screeched to a halt and after going through police Officers who wanted to confirm who she was, she ran to the side of the boy. They both hugged and, for the first time, I saw the boy cry.

"I'm sorry, mamma," he told her between sniffles. "I didn't mean to get the clothes dirty."

Although she was visibly shaken by all that was happening around her, she also seemed to know the fright her son had been in and how his actions had probably saved the lives of her family this night.

She rose from kneeling at her son's side and started to move towards the back bedroom. An Officer stopped her.

"Mam'," he stated. "I can't let you go back there. They're still processing the body."

"Well," she stated, with the firmness but kindness only a Mom would know. "Those are my little girls back there and you'd better get a way to get me back there."

Both Officer and Mom stood, not moving.

Finally, the Officer directed her how to step around the dead man in her hallway so as to not disturb the crime scene and she made her way back to her two young daughters.

She stood at the door for a minute and watched them sleep. My partner, who had been on the other side of the body, put his hand on her shoulder.

"They've been asleep through the whole thing," he said. She turned towards him. "And they have not been harmed in any way."

Mom walked into the room, touched each girl, made sure that all of the parts were in their right place and that there was no blood. She turned and walked back to John, who remained at the door. Her face turned from worry to a slight smile.

"You have one brave boy there," John continued. "I don't know how all of this will turn out but it looks like he saved them from something terrible."

Mom turned all of the way towards John and collapsed in his arms, crying hard for a moment. The boy heard her crying out front and immediately got up and started towards her.

"I really am sorry Mom!" he yelled. "We can wash that all out. I'll do it. Promise."

She left Johns arms and walked the same way back to her son, who appeared to stand a little taller to her than when she had left earlier. They both hugged and cried again.

At that one time in space, the air we were standing in, changed. Mom, realizing that this little boy probably saved the lives of her two daughters (his sisters) as well as his life (and possibly hers if she had been at home), understood the seriousness of it all – and, in the blink of an eye, she realized the true love he had for his sisters.

"I love you so much," she said with a voice that spoke a truth only a child would know from his mother. She calmed him down, assuring him that he was not in trouble.

We stood around for a minute while everyone took their role. The cops were becoming background as the Detectives arrived, the medical examiner had arrived and was writing in a large book, charting and figuring. They would be there for hours and we were not needed.

As my partner and I returned to our Ambulance, we stopped and looked back.

While it was true, that is was a typical shift, and that the house was a plain, small, regular type of house, the events that happened that evening would change a few lives forever. One was me.

I never again took safety for granted. You have to remember that I was about 26 years old and at that age when nothing could happen to me. Although I wasn't crazy with danger, I never really thought about what *might* happen.

This night changed that. I was a little more cautious in dark streets, driving in unfamiliar territory and, I must admit, a little weird when I was around any delivery drivers.

Now, don't get me wrong – I love delivery folks. They are energetic and hard working. You must remember, though, that the first time I ever came in contact with one, in full uniform, he was face down, dead of a gunshot wound, following his break-in to a strangers home.

When I got home that next morning, I realized that the one place that I should be the safest, my home, was no longer the safe haven I once thought it was. That family's home, their castle, had been invaded by evil and their lives had, for one brief moment, hung on the balance of a nine year old.

That nine year old took matters into his own hand and did what he needed to do to insure the safety of his family.

Way to go, Tyson. You done good!

TECHNOLOGY

I have always told people that "technology will kill us before it makes us better." I had no idea how great technology would be in our career path when I first started.

I also didn't know how "bad" technology would be, or why, until that day in class.

In a previous chapter, I mentioned that one of my teaching gigs was at the National Fire Academy. Although my first class was my most memorable, I am afraid to say it was not due to what we taught, but what I learned – about technology and about my students.

Particularly one.

The course was an EMS special operations course with 31 students. Most of the morning is spent on housekeeping and getting to know one another, sort of setting up the learning environment.

In this particular class, we were into our first 5 minutes, barely into the "my name is" portion when one of my students got up and exited in order to take a cell call.

Technology has made our lives somewhat easier. I say "somewhat", because along with that comes the "electronic leash" which we have become so accustomed to. Most of the students are Officers, in one form or another, and all of them have the various technical devices which keep them in contact with home. We even have computers, wired to the internet, in the back of the classrooms and encourage students, if they need to, to step back during breaks and check their email.

The only thing we ask is that they be discreet; put your cell phones on silent or vibrate, step out of the classroom if you need to take a call, silence your blackberries, etc. All of the students I have ever had, have been very courteous in regards to the electronic world.

Most of us, as instructors, realize that they people have lives and that they are away for a two week period so it is not unusual for anyone to go outside to get a message or take a call from home.

Shortly after the student had gotten up and walked into the hallway, I looked out to find him still talking on a cell phone and motioning me outside.

His face looked strange and I asked my co-instructor to take the class as I exited. When I got to him, I realized he was shaking and conversing on his cell, talking in short sentences and listening intently to whomever was talking.

He looked up with tears in his eyes. "They're doing CPR on my wife right now," he said, visibly shaken.

Ah, technology. Did I say it was supposed to make life easier? Of course it is! I remember when I was younger, we had pagers that were so big, it would dig into your side and cause bruising and couldn't hear beyond a 3 mile radius of the radio tower.

Someday, people would tell me, we will all have computers in our homes. Who were they kidding? The first real computer I had ever seen filled a 30 by 30 foot room at a major University. Who would want that in their home?

They went on to tell me that one day we would have some type of "radio" phone that we could stand anywhere and talk to anyone in the world. The phone currently at my home weighed as much as my shoes and was tethered by a thick black wire. Were they pulling my leg?

No, they were not. Today, we sure as hell have technology. We could hear from the boss, no matter where you, or they, were. Dispatch could now page you on a box smaller than your watch (and some were watches) - even if we are showering (or doing any number of other bodily functions).

And now, – now, I was watching technology that was *too* good, bringing news live, as it happened, to a husband who was listening to the sounds of his wife's life slip away.

"Do you have the monitor on her yet?" he asked.

There was an answer. Silence from the student.

"No, no, she was sick this weekend but had felt better on Sunday," he said, explaining her history. "No, no medical history whatsoever. She doesn't take any meds."

I looked into his eyes and realized that he knew the seriousness of what was occurring. He was a seasoned Paramedic and a Fire Chief from a large town in the Northeast. He knew the percentage of patients who live from cardiac arrest. He knew the probability of his wife living through this critical time. He knew – we would all have known – and yet, he hung onto the chance of, "what if they got there in time? *Please,* let them have gotten there in time….."

He leaned over to me. "The Paramedic who is working on my wife is one of mine." As a chief Officer, I understand the pride we take in our employees.

I don't know why he told me that.

The people on the other end of the telephone told him they were going to continue working and transport her to the Hospital. They suggested that he get home. He agreed and hung up.

We stood in the hallway for a minute. I asked for her name. "Jenny", he said. I silently prayed that Jenny would be OK.

"My son is in the military," he told me. "He's in Japan. I've got to get ahold of him."

I went back into class to tell my other instructor what had occurred and that I was going to get the student started on the path home.

While class continued, I and the student walked upstairs to the administrative offices of the academy. Being my first day, I didn't even know who to go to, so I went to the person who was my contact for my travel.

Judy was at her desk when I told her the news. It was as if a switch had been pulled in the area where we were at.

She asked if he was staying on campus (some students didn't) and he confirmed he was. She looked at me and realized how new I was.

"Don, why don't you walk him over to the dorm so we can start the checkout process," she said with as calm a voice I had ever heard coming from a non-responder person. "I'll start booking flights and get him a ride to the airport from here.

We left and walked across campus. He kept pulling out his phone, not dialing, just looking at it.

Although we didn't talk, I could feel the helplessness he was carrying. He was hundreds of miles away and couldn't do anything but pray. I think he and I both silently did that on the two block walk to the dorm.

When we arrived, the front desk folks already had the news and had the forms ready. He went to his room to pack and I stood, looking at the various pictures hanging in the lobby.

I picked up the phone and dialed home.

"Hi sweetie," I said. Barbara new something was wrong and asked if I was ok.

I explained what was going on and I just wanted to call and tell her how much I loved her. We both spoke for the moment but, to this day, I can't remember what it was about.

I saw the student coming back to the lobby with two suitcases and I hung up, going up to the desk and making sure all paperwork was in order. Two signatures and he was clear.

The silent walk back to the office was different. He looked up to me.

"They called," he said. "They called the code about 10 minutes ago."

At that moment, the sadness, the fear, the realization that what I said to others – *make sure you say goodbye each time you leave your loved ones. You never know if they're coming back* – took on a real meaning.

I don't mean that the way it sounds. I know that's reality. I saw it every day in the streets. And, yet, I had never been so close to someone who had lived it.

He left home yesterday, on the way to a two week class at the NFA. 24 hours later, his wife was dead.

We got to the office and Judy told him she had three different tickets on hold, depending how he wanted to get home. A volunteer driver was on the way in to get the van and would get him to the airport quickly.

He and I hugged and I asked him if he had gotten hold of the Red Cross. He said he had called but they needed some documentation but were working on it. I told him he and his family would be in our prayers. I left and went back to class.

Downstairs, the students were starting to take notes on the background information we gave in the first three days. They all stopped and looked up at me when I entered.

"How is he?" they almost said in unison.

"They called the code a few minutes ago," I told them. You could tell that the entire class felt the pain and sorrow. *He was one of us.*

I mentioned to them how the process worked and that the NFA had a wonderful program of making sure emergencies were a top priority. Whatever they had heard about bureaucracy in the Federal system, that certainly didn't apply here.

I asked if we could say a prayer for him and his family. Everyone bowed their heads.

After the class, I wanted to find out what happened but, you know how life gets in the way. I returned to work and put the class behind me.

One year later, at a special operations class, Don, my co-instructor and I, were waiting for the students to get out of orientation. In walked my student.

"How are you doing?" I asked and we both hugged. For a moment, we both had tears in our eyes.

"I'm ok," he stated. "One day at a time."

"Did your son make it home?" I asked, remembering how worried he was.

"He sure did," he said. "The Red Cross folks were wonderful"/

"So," I stated. "What are you doing here?"

He smiled. "She would have wanted me to finish," he said. He said it with a small voice and a big heart. I can't explain how it sounded but it was pure love.

I smiled. "Let's get you a seat."

THE BRIDGE

They probably never met, these two passengers on a Greyhound bus. They had never nodded or smiled or even made eye contact. They had, after all, no mutual friends, no shared interests. He was 20, an exceptional college student, on the school tennis team, standing on the brink of his life. She was 92, stiffening with advanced arthritis, planning another trip to her native Sweden, undoubtedly the last given her growing physical limitations. They had nothing in common at all.

Except, as they settled into their Greyhound bus seats, heading south under gray and threatening skies, they were about to die together.

....

My part time job involved working as the EMS Director for a local helicopter company, which, among other things, did helicopter Ambulance runs from an out of county Hospital to our trauma/cardiac center. There were, at the time, no facility transfer helicopter services and only one "on-scene" Hospital ship, in Pensacola, FL.

We carried large, wallet size pagers with us that were one way, VHF and usually hard to hear. I heard mine go off at 7:50.

"Don, come to the office ASAP, Don." I could tell it was Gwen, the owner's, daughter's voice.

Strange, I thought. Usually, she asked me to call to get the info on where we were picking the patient up and where we were going to (usually, always to our facility). I called anyhow.

"Don," she yelled into the phone, a very noisy background almost drowning her out. "The skyway bridge has fallen into the water and they need all medical help they can get. They have asked 79 Tango to respond."

79 Tango was our call sign but we had *never* gone on an emergent run. I got dressed and drove to the hanger.
…………………………..
At 7:25 a.m. on May 9, 1980, with the Greyhound approaching Pinellas Point a few miles from the north end of the Sunshine Skyway bridge, Capt. John Lerro tensed at the helm of the freighter Summit Venture, a ship as long as two football fields. Lerro, 37, an experienced harbor pilot from Tampa, shouldered the responsibility of guiding the Summit Venture from the Gulf of Mexico 58.4 miles up Tampa Bay to the Port of Tampa. It is one of the longest shipping channels in the world, and one of the most treacherous, given the shallow waters of the Bay and the ambush style of Florida weather. With the ship's belly empty of cargo and her tanks nearly empty of ballast, she rode high in the water. She ran through intermittent fog and rain along the first 19 miles of her journey. Then southwest winds exploded to tropical-storm force. Rain sheeted at rates exceeding 7 inches an hour. Visibility plunged to near zero, and shipboard radar failed. It couldn't have happened at a worse point. Lerro faced the most critical course change of the run, a 13-degree turn that would take him between the two main piers of the Skyway Bridge. It was at almost this exact spot that the Coast Guard cutter Blackthorn had been rammed four months

earlier by the tanker Capricorn. The Blackthorn sank. Twenty-three men died.

Lerro approached the critical bend on a ship weighing nearly 20,000 tons battered by winds of nearly 60 mph. And, he approached it blind.

……………..

The 20 minute drive to the hanger was treacherous. Rain looked like a solid sheet of water. I had to slow to 20 MPH due to the heaviness of the storm. It was pouring just that bad at the hanger. *We're not going up in this weather*, I thought.

When I got there, it was as if the sky had fallen in. I had to park in the street because the parking lot was full of TV vans. I couldn't see the front of the office from the street.

The small lobby was filled with reporters and camera folks, all clamoring on when the "next chopper" was headed out there. I heard one coming into the pad, followed by the engine dying down and Mike, our best (and craziest) pilot coming in, scowl on his face, with three reporters following.

"But, you've got to get us out there," they yelled. "We'll pay double - triple!"

"I can't see the ground," Mike yelled. "We are grounded!"

As the reporters followed him around the lobby, shouting out totally outrageous amounts of money, I went into the back, unnoticed. There, I found Ray loading up the ship.

"Did you hear?" he asked

"The skyway bridge?" I asked.
"Yeah, a ship hit it and a fourth of a mile segment has gone into the sea" he continued. "They think a bus went over along with several cars."

The rain seemed to let up and then, it suddenly stopped.

"Let's roll her out," Ray said.
………………..
Anthony Gattus he didn't like what he saw at all. "It was a lousy day to start with," Gattus recalled. "It started raining hard 2 or 3 miles before we got to the Skyway. It got really dark. I don't like rain and cold and darkness. Didn't then. Don't now."

Gattus, now 81, was a passenger in a yellow Buick headed south with three other men to ferry cars back for sale in Pinellas County. Richard Hornbuckle, the owner of the Buick, was behind the wheel. Jim Crispin sat beside Hornbuckle in the front seat. Kenneth Holmes sat beside Gattus in back.

"Hornbuckle was a real good driver," Gattus said. "I always felt safe with him.

When the rain started hard, Hornbuckle slowed way down. Twenty. Don't think he could have been going faster than 20 mph.

"I remember a blue pickup passed us." Gattus said. "I remember a bus passed us." We stopped when we realized we had run out of bridge in the middle of the bridge."

……………..

We grabbed the tail of the aircraft and, with its wheels on the skids, moved it out to the pad.

"Let's go," Ray said, it a hurrying kind of voice.

As I plugged the starter cart into the aircraft (batteries were expensive so we always used a cart when we were at home), a reporter came out onto the pad, a clear safety violation.

"Hey, where are they going?" he yelled. "Can't we go with them?"

The Manager came out and pulled him back into the office. He looked mad.

…………………..

On the water below, Lerro considered his options. Visibility was so bad he could no longer see the bow of his ship. He judged it too risky to turn the Summit Venture out of the shipping channel to the north to anchor and ride out the storm because the outbound Pure Oil had been approaching. Without radar or visibility to locate the tanker, Lerro feared he might ram her if he steered across her path. If he tried to stop, or if he turned south out of the channel, the winds could usurp control of the ship and hurl him into the bridge.

Thinking the wind was still from the southwest (his right), Lerro judged it would push the Summit Venture safely through the main spans of the Skyway. He made the decision to proceed. Lerro didn't know the squall had forced the wind around to the west-northwest (his left). Instead of keeping him in the channel, it pushed his high-riding vessel off course.

At 7:32, the weather cleared marginally. Lerro saw part of the bridge superstructure directly ahead. With heart stopping clarity, he realized he was no longer in the shipping channel. He ordered a series of maneuvers, including emergency reversal of the engines and the deployment of the anchors. But it was too late. At 7:33, the bow of the Summit Venture collided with bridge pier 2S. The pier toppled, taking the roadway with it.
………………………………..
We cleared through the tower, now being *lifeguard 79 tango*, a radio designation that we were on the way to an emergency response.

As we approached the causeway, we looked out towards the Skyway.

The bridge, completed in 1987, was a centerpiece for Tampa Bay. All boats that came into the Bay passed under it. Hundreds of pictures have been taken of it, with and without a sunrise. At the time, it was one of the longest bridges in Florida.

We couldn't see anything other than the normal span. As we turned to the left, it became apparent, something was missing.

The far, sea-side lanes of the bridge seemed off. As we got closer, it was apparent that a portion of the bridge, the far side, was missing.

I remember the larger portion of the bridge, looking as if it was barely hanging on, with a car, precariously perched on the end. As we circled over the top, it appeared there was a man at that car, trying to get something out of his trunk. A set of golf clubs appeared and the piece of the bridge he was standing on continued to swing in the wind as if barely attached.

We turned back north towards an LZ that had been set up. That's when I saw it.

Lying on its side, looking as if someone with large scissors had cut off the top of it, lay a greyhound bus, without its top side. As I refocused my eyes, I realized there were bodies floating on the top of the water.

This was very bad.

We approached a parking area where another aircraft had landed. It was a local TV station and we both wondered how they had gotten here so fast. The rain was very bad and it would have been suicide for any pilot to try to fly through it.

We landed and walked over to a Sheriff's vehicle.

"We're with Suncoast Helicopters and have an air Ambulance if you need it," Ray announced.

The several police Officers around the car looked up without an expression and simply stared. One walked over to Ray.

"Everyone's dead," he said, matter of fact. "No survivors," and, with that, he turned back to the car to look at various maps on the hood.

Ray and I walked over the edge of the water and looked out. The water was very calm and somewhat pretty. The span of the North bound side stood proudly.

The span of the Southbound, however, looked wounded. It looked like someone had shredded it. We could see some metal sticking up from the bottom of the water under the damaged span.

Next to the 2nd span was a very big ship. It appeared that a portion of the bridge had fallen onto the front of the bridge, still intact and with a pick-up truck sitting on the cut-off roadway.

"I guess the boat hit it," Ray said.

From our angle, we could no longer see the greyhound bus, or the various cars at the bottom of the channel. We could see several bodies floating near the bridge. There was a smaller law enforcement boat there trying to bring those bodies up onto their deck.
As we started to walk back to our ship, we met the TV pilot.

"How did you get here so quick?" Ray asked him, tilting his hat in a greeting to the other pilot.

"My boss ordered me to fly here and I did," he said. "News waits for no one."

Ray was dumbfounded. "You're PIC (Pilot in Command) and you make those calls. I would have never flown in that weather."

"That's because you don't work for TV", the other pilot answered. "I am given the choice every day. Fly there or be fired."

Ray walked up to him and got real close to his face.

"Never," he told the TV pilot.

In a blink of an eye, 35 people ceased to exist and the lives of their families had changed forever. A mistake made by a ship captain 1,000 feet below the road surface had changed their destiny and the lives of many who witnessed the collapse.

Today, I don't see many Greyhound buses, but when I do, I remember the day the bridge fell, the day many got in too big of a hurry and how everyone's life who was involved, was changed forever.

The Wedding Dress

I saw the wedding dress, almost immediately upon getting out of my truck.

I first noticed how white it was – and how soiled it was, all at the same time.

I had to look for a minute before I realized that the dress surrounded a body. What was left of the bride lay face down and motionless.

What was I doing here?

………..

In the days before smaller and smaller cell phones, we were issued what we loving called "bricks", large battery powered cell phones and mine rang early on a Sunday morning, around 3 AM.

"This is dispatch," the voice said. "They've got a body out on the interstate that they really have to get off the ground ASAP."

That wasn't terribly unusual. We had been transporting the bodies for the Coroner, in his van, for some time, helping their office out and keeping an Ambulance from being used. In a small rural area, resources are scarce.

So, my Assistant Director and I took turns at body duty. It is not as easy as it sounds.

The van is plain, no marking, with one of our stretchers in the back and appropriate gear for such a task – body bags, gloves, some cleaner. The Coroner would call us when one needed transporting to the morgue. We usually met volunteer firefighters on scene who helped us load the body and the Hospital staff met us at the other end to help us unload.

Although it sounds gruesome, it is a needed service. *Someone* has to get the body to the proper place so that the grieving process can begin. They are as much of a patient as the live ones in the Ambulance.

And, yet, this one was very, very different.

Death scenes have a hue to them. I don't know if I can explain it but I'll try.

Death happens, quite frankly, when the body either quits working from age, health or an unnatural event happens. Those unnatural things can be auto accidents, shootings, stabbings……you get my drift.

When we arrive in the body van, everyone in law enforcement knows who we are and what we are there to do. Most of the civilians, either standing outside the house or near the wreck, do not. We do not wear any identification but do appear in a professional golf-type shirt. We like to think of that part of the job as starting the healing process.

Most think it's pretty disgusting.

And, here, tonight, along the interstate, in the silence of a rural night, with the stars above us and a beautiful almost-full moon standing overhead, I started to realize that someone's life that had hours before just begun on a grand adventure, had tragically ended.

As I stood beside the van door, I could plainly see that the patient was wearing a long, flowing white dress. Even with her face down, you could tell it was a wedding dress.

"Hey," the deputy yelled. I looked over at him, standing on the other side of the service road.

"Over here," he said. His voice was flat, although most scenes like this rarely carry any emotion. It simply gets in the way of the job.

I grabbed the stretcher from the back of the van and started to roll it over towards the deputy. I didn't understand at first, as the woman in the white flowing dress was in the other direction. As I approached the deputy, my eyes went down and to the right. I couldn't see him at first and then, I realized he was there.

A young man, maybe in his 20's (I have always been bad at guessing deceased patients ages), dressed in a black suit, possibly a tux, also face down. There was mud on the suit, as if his entire body had skidded along the highway for some distance.

"Wedding?" I asked. The deputy looked very concerned.

"Yeah," he said. "You saw the bride, right?"

I nodded.

"Very sad," he continued. "Probably married a few hours ago, out of State, driving through to get to their honeymoon."

"Geez, they didn't even have time to change", he whispered.

I went over to the patient and turned him away from me so I could see his face. He looked like a teenager, asleep on the ground – except for the horrific cut on his face and the obvious trauma to his neck.

I was sure it was snapped in two.

I looked over my shoulder at the other body, in that pristine white dress, lying across the road in the same face-down position of her new husband.

I stood back up for a minute and simply stood still in the night. The night seemed unusually quiet, even for a rural area. Usually, in the late fall, you can hear the katydids and crickets, maybe some dog barking or other noise.

Tonight, there was nothing.

The landscape was somewhat surreal. An exit on an interstate, a car on its roof and two people, dressed in formal attire, both dead. They had just started their lives in a ceremony that I am sure was glorious. Their lives ended in an unceremonious way, although the crash probably looked stupendous, if horrific.

In my career, I have seen people whose life ended in the strangest of ways. The normal, "they didn't wake up" death, the "he's not my husband" uncomfortable hotel room death, the "found hung in his parent's bedroom" death. I even attended a cardiac arrest for a father who, while dancing with his bride, dropped on the dance floor.

While some might see death as depressing or gruesome, I have come to realize that death is the same as birth, only in the reverse. As babies are born, people die. I have to admit that those who are, for example, dancing with their daughter or working in a career field they love, die as I believe they would want to: doing what they love. I often felt that, when the day comes for my exit from this stage, I am sitting behind a desk looking at fuel bills, I will have cheated myself. Dying while treating a patient, helping someone out of a crushed car or holding someone's hand during a medical emergency, while it would be tragic, would be exactly where I would want to be.

Not to be consumed with work, should my demise happen after work is finished and I have retired (according to friends, I then become twice as busy as when at work), I hope the day arrives when I am scuba diving, riding on my brothers Jet Ski (sorry Walker, but I promise not to crash it when it happens) or White Water Rafting in Colorado. I want to keep moving, keep investing in my life, keep living.

Sitting on the interstate, I look over at the bride and then look at the groom. I look back at the bride – that image cannot leave my head.

They both loved each other enough to commit the rest of their lives together. They didn't know that time would be so short.

That's really the moral of the story; we think we have time but, under our breath, we admit to ourselves we do not.

Living life, realizing that it could end while you are reading this, helps us all to understand how precious life is – and how we should live each day as if it were our last.

As I thought of that, I looked up again.

I saw the wedding dress. It was so white. In the darkness of the interstate exit, it was almost shimmering.

I bet that was what he thought when he first saw her walking down the aisle.

I took the stretcher from the body van and went to work, getting the couple to their next resting place.

STORIES

Almost everyone I meet asks me for the "grossest" call I've ever been on.

Trust me, I have plenty – and usually have a few on deck when someone asks. They rarely ask for the most amazing call, or the call in which you saved a life.

I don't know what this fascination is that we have with horror. I know when I actually ran those "bad" calls, most often, I was either panicked or sick to my stomach while we were running the call and, more often than not, the smell or site remained in my nostrils or brain for days or weeks after.

So, it is rare that when someone asks for my worst call, I actually start with that one: Instead, I tell them something that happened that was funny or cute.

Besides, no one could *possibly* get the grossness of any call by simply telling the story.

As I mentioned earlier, many of them, in fact, too many, have sights and smells and feels that don't go away from when you had them and can't be transferred to the receiver in a story.

Some of the stories I have made into separate chapters in this book, either because they tell an important story, give a life-saving lesson, or simply sit in my head, either as one of the amazing times, or one of the horrors. Both swim around in my head and, on occasion, give me a smile or an all-night nightmare.

The following are short stories about life on the streets as I remember them.

. . . .

We pulled up to what appeared to be a one car accident, the car in a ditch, on its side, with volunteer firefighters all about, yelling and waving us over to the ladder that went to the top (or the right side when it was in its proper position) of the car.

A firefighter at the top told me there were two elderly folks inside and they were covered in something terrible.

"Blood", my first thought. I got halfway up the ladder and a female's hand came out of the top for the car reach for something or someone. I remember she was screaming.

I reached over, without looking, and noted immediately that her hand was covered in – well, ooze. It was clear, it smelled bad and I didn't know what it was, but knew it could be fluid from her brain.

You see, they teach us that if someone is bleeding from the ear, we should take the corner of a sterile bandage (often called a 4X4) and dip it into the blood. If it was fluid from her brain, it would separate itself on the bandage. Should we see that, we would realize she had a very serious brain injury.

I pulled my hand back and smelled. It smelled bad. She kept screaming at the top of her lungs.

It was very hard to concentrate when they screamed like that.

As I reached the top of the car, I looked in and found an 80-something woman, hanging by her seat belt (something not in every car at the time) and pushing on her husband, who was all the way down in the well of the left side of the sideways car.

I pulled my hand out and smelled it. It smelled terrible and I was afraid it was my first look at Cerebra-spinal fluid. This is the fluid that surrounds your brain and your spinal cord. If you had a little bit coming out of your ears, it was a sign of a serious brain injury. If a patient had it all over their blouse - - Well, I couldn't imagine what that would indicate but I was pretty sure it was serious.

As I talked to her, I asked all the questions we were supposed to ask to ascertain her injuries. She wouldn't answer but just continued screaming. It didn't appear she had any injuries, less the fluid all over her front. When she finally stopped screaming, she said her hip hurt, from the seat belt. Eventually, we found her to be awake, alert, oriented X 3 (person, place and time), had no lacerations, no fractures (as far as we could tell) and only this slime all over the front of her.

Then, I saw it; on the bottom of the car (actually lying on the left driver's door) was a two and ½ dozen egg carrier, empty. As I looked around, I realized that were at least two and ½ dozen eggs broken in the car, much of which ended up on the front of my patient's dress. I do remember her mentioning how upset she was that, if she lived through this, she would have to go buy a new plat of eggs.

I moved my hand to my nose again and took another sniff. Even though I knew now that the fluid on my hands was not her brains leaking out of a devastating skull fracture, it made no difference. I would, from that point on, associate that smell with a hemorrhage in the brain.

Later in my life, I would start a diet of egg beaters, some for their health but mostly because I still couldn't stand the smell of raw eggs.

. . . .

As I sat in the dispatch control center (i.e., a room smaller than your bedroom with one dial telephone and one tube-powered two-way radio), I noticed how quiet it had been.

That spells trouble in this business, whether you say it or even think it.

The radio lit up.

"Unit 61 to base," Lorenzo called.

"Go head 61," Larry answered, rolling his eyes. He knew there were no calls on the board – so what could it be?

"61, is there someone in headquarters who reads short-hand?" he asked.

We looked at each other. Neither of us knew.

We looked through the small door into the office and wondered. We knew Ms. Mary, the queen of the office, probably knew all there was to know about anything office-like. Short-hand? We weren't sure.

"Stand by," Larry said in as official a voice as I had ever heard.

He asked me to go find out and I left the command center and walked into the front office.

Funny, these women had all been there for years and, yet, even with the command center only 40 feet away, we never talked, never inter-mingled on the days' events. They were billing, we were operations.

"Ms. Mary," I asked in a softer voice than I used in operations.

"What is it Don?" all with a smile. It was like talking to one's mother.

"Do you know how to read short-hand?"

She looked at me odd. "Why?" she wondered.

"Well, I don't know", I answered her. "A crew on the street wanted to know."

She got a curious look on her face. "I have been printing and reading shorthand for over 30 years," he stated. "I don't know why an Ambulance driver would need to know that."

She got up with me as we both went into the operations section and she followed me into the command center.

"Larry," I said. Ms. Mary knows shorthand. She's curious why Lorenzo would ask."

"Lorenzo?" she coughed. "No telling what that crazy boy wants." It's obvious she knew the crews as well as us too.

"Unit 61, this is base," Larry called out.

"Go head for 61," a voice said.

"Just curious," Larry stated, "What do you need that for?"

"Base," Lorenzo stated. "Police here have a homeless guy arrested and he has a bunch of notes on what looks like a steno-pad and they think it might be stolen. It looks like shorthand and we are just around the corner from base, so they asked me and I asked you."

Seemed simple enough. Ms. Mary was somewhat excited, suddenly in the world of the street, deciphering who knew what.

"Unit 61," Larry told them. "Ms. Mary can read and decipher shorthand."

Silence.

"Copy base," Lorenzo finally said. We expected either Lorenzo or the cops to show up within a few minutes.

The radio hummed once again.

"Base, ready to copy?" Lorenzo said.

Copy what? What was he talking about? We both looked at each other again, and then to Ms. Mary. We had no idea where this was going with this.

Larry looked at me and shrugged his shoulders. "Go head 61."

"Ok," Lorenzo stated. "The first one looks like a backwards Q, then an upside down W, a smaller squiggle line with a slash in it, another upside down W…….."

Ms. Mary looked ticked. Larry looked like he was going to bust out laughing.

"Unit 61," he interrupted the unit. "I think you have to bring that by for us to see it." He had a chuckle under his breath.

Lorenzo was not to be undaunted.

"Then, it looks like a sideways b with a small dot on the top of it," he continued. "I don't even know what to call the next symbol, possibly a soccer ball with a stick through it and a small dog collar with an arrow at the top."

By now, other units were clicking their mikes (in the VHF world that was code for laughter) and Larry and I were laughing and Lorenzo continued his "read" of the code.

When we stopped laughing, we noticed that Ms. Mary had already left and gone back into the office.

I am not sure if she thought we were in on it or not, but I am sure she was pretty disgusted with all of it. I don't think I ever saw her back in operations again.

....

Responding to a downed truck driver, we realized our address was the County dump.

It was a large complex, one which the general public rarely saw. This was *the* dump, where rumor had it they had buried one of the dead elephants from the zoo. Everything from Foley bags, to rotting food, to plastic to paper, to – well, everything that goes to the dump – was buried there (or about to be).

This time, it was quite different.

At the gate, a pick-up truck met us and led us into the bowels of the dump. As we went through the gate, we realized that *we* hadn't even seen the inside of the dump –

most patients were brought to us at the gate and we treated them from that point.

The first thing you notice is the obvious smell. It is absolutely gagging. It had been raining most of the night and that morning, so the clay they used had gotten quite wet and, when driving, spun up into the Ambulance.

Lovely.

We go to the top of the pit and as we came over the ridge, we stopped, realizing that our large truck would never be able to make it back up from the bottom of the pit. We decided to park there and walk down.

As we approached the bottom, we recognized a garbage truck, with its loader in the up position. It was apparent that it had dumped its load, but had not gone down.

Three men stood around the pile as we approached. No one was talking – that was always a bad sign.

As we approached the pile of garbage looking to have come from the truck, I looked down at my feet and realized my shiny street shoes were covered in the muck of the dump. I looked back at our unit, freshly washed for the morning, and saw chunks of clay and garbage stuck to the sides and in the wheel wells. It was going to take a steam cleaner to get rid of the stink.

The smell of garbage reeked everywhere and I saw that the mud had come on the cuffs of my pants. I was sure I was going to have to get rid of these shoes. I hoped we weren't near the dead elephant.

I suddenly heard what sounded like a gunshot and a whistling, overhead, like an incoming round. I instinctively ducked behind the Ambulance.

"Damn birds," one of the Supervisors said. He had a type of gun in his hand. We both starred at him.

"If you don't do that every few minutes, the birds will carry you away," he shouted. I relaxed from my crouching position behind the unit.

That's when I saw them.

As I looked towards the pile, where the three men were staring – I saw the legs of what I assumed to be one of their co-workers.

They were not moving.

As I approached them, one of the Supervisors told me that Mr. Dead garbage (not his real name) had been unable to get a portion of jammed garbage out of his truck and, as they so many times told them not to do, reached up and attempted to pull the jam out.

The resulting action buried him in his own garbage.

There he was, buried from his knees forward. His hat had fallen off of his head and lay next to his right foot.

"Well?" the Supervisor asked.

"Well," I said. "We need to get the Coroner. Don't move anything."

The complaints started from the men, how this was going to put them way behind schedule and that they couldn't put garbage anywhere else for that day, due to preparations, etc. The humanity of a life lost seemed to be reduced to efficiency of the dump.

"Hey," one of the three co-workers said to me.

"Hey," I said. After all, what do you say to the guy whose partner was just buried in garbage?

"Do you think he'd mind if I took his boots?"

You've got to be kidding me.

"I don't think you should remove anything until the Coroner gets here," I said. I was trying to be nice, yet official. After all, this could be a close friend of his. I didn't want to seem uncaring.

"Oh," he said, somewhat disappointed.

"What about his hat? Do you think he'd mind if I took his hat?"

"DON'T TOUCH ANYTHING," I said, forcefully now.

I was sure that if we hadn't been there, the Coroner would have found a naked man from the knees down (and from the neck up).

All of us, EMS, co-workers, Supervisors, stood in the garbage looking at the man buried in his work.

It took us an entire shift to steam clean the undercarriage of the Ambulance until the smell of garbage stopped drifting into the patient compartment.

And, for the record, when we left, he still had his boots on.

And, no, we never found the elephant.

…………..

"Unit 61, base" the dispatcher drowned over the radio.

Larry was a very laid back dispatcher, but as sharp as a tack. You couldn't do that job without knowing where everything was, where everyone was, and what the shortest way was to get there.

Larry knew all of that. He also had that relaxed, "so-what-if-your-pants-are-on-fire" voice. If you were panicked, it was his job to talk you back off of the cliff. He did that with style and was always protective of his co-workers.

"Unit 61 is at 30th and Fletcher," the EMT answered.

Lee, one of the more seasoned veterans, was also a straight professional. He knew his medicine and was caring towards all of his patients. That would include those who pointed out that he was Jewish, sometimes not in the most flattering ways.

It was his *voice* that always got people. Although, as I said, he was the most compassionate, his voice, in person, was comforting and caring. On the radio, however, he always sounded like he didn't give a damn.

Larry looked at the mic, reacting to Lee's less-than-caring sound. "You left some equipment at the ER," he said.

What he was talking about, Lee thought. He had secured and cleaned all equipment. How could he say that on the radio for everyone to hear? *It wasn't his equipment,* he thought.

Larry, waiting for an answer to his statement, was hoping he wouldn't ask *what* equipment was missing.

About 3 minutes before this radio transmission, a Nurse at the ER had called and asked if Unit 61 had just left there.

"Yeah, they just went enroute back to Brandon," he told the Nurse.

"Well," she said, laughing under her breath. "You need to get them back here. A citizen just came in with their stretcher and it's got their unit number on it. He said it flew right out of the back and into the intersection as they were turning."

Larry prayed – *please don't ask me what kind of equipment.*

"Unit 60," Lee said in a drone. "We have all of our equipment."

That was what Larry was afraid of. Sometimes, we EMTs do get a sort of pre-Madonna attitude and, in those days, the VHF radio allowed everyone to hear everything. An item like leaving your clipboard or monitor behind could ride you for weeks.

"Unit 60," Larry tried one more time. "Please go back to the ER and see Sally. She'll explain it."

Frustrated, Lee knew they had not forgotten anything and he wanted to get back to their district. They were far outside of their response area and response times, particularly in rural Brandon, were not the best they could be when they were gone.

"Unit 61," Lee said, now ticked. "What equipment do they have?"

Well, that was it. The cards had been called and Larry had no exit except to tell them, and the whole world, what had happened.

"Unit 61," Larry said, in as straight a voice as he could, never a hard problem for him. "Your stretcher fell out of your Ambulance and a citizen recovered it and took it to the ER."

Lee suddenly turned around and, in a shoulder-slouching motion, turned back to his partner and told him that their stretcher was missing.

"It can't be ours," his partner said. "I put it in myself."

"Well," Lee said to him. "Apparently, you didn't secure it. It's gone."

Larry, in the meantime, was waiting for them to answer their intention. They couldn't get in for all of the "clicking" on the radio.

Radio microphone "clicking" continued from others who were, no doubt, laughing with us (or at us, who knew).

"Unit 61, you copy?" Larry asked.

"61 copies, enroute to the ER".

Red faced and somewhat mad at each other, both returned to the ER to retrieve their stretcher.

For the rest of the day, they were asked by everyone they met, some they knew and others they didn't, whether they remembered their stretcher.

Embarrassing.

. . . .

We pulled up to the house in Ybor City. Parked in the front were the Rescue unit and a fire truck. At that time, Rescue was the only system that had Paramedics. They usually didn't have a fire engine go with them unless they needed the manpower. To see one at a house at this early hour was not a good sign, after all, it was 2:45 AM.

Outside, it seemed rather quiet. All of the neighbors had not heard the commotion, most likely because, at that time, we didn't like to make a lot of noise at night. Nosy neighbors generally got in the way and, although they really weren't being nosy but were concerned for their neighbors, it was better if we could keep them in their beds.

So, the outside was somewhat serene. Rescue and the engine, idling outside, along with our Ambulance, was all you could hear.

Inside was another story.

As we entered the front door, we could hear it. A firefighter, counting CPR compressions and, after every 5th compression, the resuscitator would swoosh it's oxygen.

We turned the corner to see the medics working on a young 50ish male who had been taken from the bed to the floor so that CPR could be done on a hard surface. IV bags were up and running, empty drug boxes were strewn everywhere, the Captain of the crew called out.

"Another Epi,"he yelled. The third person, usually used as a scribe, wrote it down. Epinephrine was another word for

Adrenaline, which was given every 10 minutes to every cardiac arrest, in the hopes of stimulating the heart.

"Clear," he yelled. His hands were holding the paddles to the patient's chest and you could hear the defibrillator charging up.

Everyone held their hands above their heads, as if it was custom to show that you were no longer touching the patient.

"Clear, clear, everybody clear," came the final call from the Captain.

The defibrillator discharged. The patent slightly jumped.

Everyone looked at the scope.

There was a beat. Then two, then several.

"Check for a pulse," he ordered. I reached over towards the man's groin to see if I could feel a femoral pulse.

"I've got a pulse and it in line with the scope," I said, smiling.

I can't tell you what the feeling is when that happens. At that time, it didn't happen that often and, when it did, it was like a home run, like a touchdown at the 2 second mark. Everyone took ownership of it, even if you were only the one holding the IV bag or writing down drug dosages.

"Ok," he said, looking at us. "Let's get him moving."

While all of us make sure that the wires, IV tubes, airways and such were clear as we started to move him to a board and then to our stretcher, I heard the Captain ask his wife where she wanted him to go.

I heard it, in that typical Cuban drawl. "Augusto Centiva," was her answer.

Augusto Centiva was a membership-only Spanish Hospital in the Ybor City area that had a one bed emergency room. They had a Doctor Carbona who lived there and was the "resident Doctor."

AC was not a Hospital in which you wanted to take a critical patient. Although the people there were very friendly and patient centered, they simply weren't staffed or equipped for critical patients.

"Ma'am," the captain replied. "I would recommend TGH since he is so sick. We can move him to Augusto Hospital after he's stabilized.

The wife raised her voice and demanded AC. They were members and that was a wonderful community Hospital and we were going there. Period.

The Captain looked back at us. The patient had been secured and was still not breathing. A firefighter bagged him every 5 second.

"Ok, boys," he said. "AC it is."

The ride to the Hospital was uneventful, except we had actually gotten someone back from the dead. He was starting to breathe on his own but we decided to keep the airway tube inserted and help him until a Doctor could look at him.

"As we pulled into the tiny driveway, we realized there was no one outside to meet us.

"Great," Captain said.

We entered the ER and directed the stretcher over to the one bed. The Nurse, leaning back in a chair and sleeping, stood up.

"What have we got here?" she asked, again in that Cuban accented lingo.

"51 year old found in cardiac arrest," the captain stated. "We've got a pulse and he has started breathing after some work."

The Nurse wasn't listening. She was on the phone to Doctor Carbona, screaming he had to get down here and it was serious.

As we continued to bag the patient, now on their bed, we tried to give the Nurse a history but she wouldn't enter the room.

We could see down the hallway and saw Dr. Carbona walking as if he was going to get ice cream. He looked like we had woke him up, disheveled, wearing a typical Doctors white coat, unbuttoned. His hair shot out in all directions and it seemed as if he was walking towards us in automatic mode.

"So, what do we have?" he asked as he entered the room. We had been there 15 minutes.

The captain started again.

"51 year old male, found in cardiac arrest at home," he stated.

"Wait"! The Doctor ordered.

Dr. Carbona reached over to his neck and felt for a pulse. The monitor beeped as each pulse happened and the patient was now almost breathing on his own.

"He's dead," the Doctor said. He pulled the sheet over the face of the patient.

The wife went down to her knees and started to scream.

"What time is it?" he asked the Nurse, wanting to know the time of death.

Before she could answer, I saw the Captain turn a deep red.

"It's time for us to get the hell out of here," he said. He pointed to us and the two firefighters who were still in the room and made a motion as if to lift the board off of the bed and back onto our stretcher.

As time seemed to stop, the good Doctor and Nurse, faces of disbelief, and the wife, with the face of hope, turned and watched as Rescue 4 and Ambulance 20 disregarded the Physicians order and placed the living patient back on their stretcher.

The Captain grabbed the wife's hand.

"Follow us if you want him to live." He said to her

As we headed out the door, the Doctor started screaming.

"You can't do that," he screamed. "I pronounced him."

"The hell you did," the captain grumbled under his breath. We loaded the patient back into the Ambulance.

"Where to?" my partner asked.

"TGH, where else?" he said. "We should have gone there in the first place."

We arrived, told them some story about why we stopped at AC, gave them the rundown and he was admitted within the hour to ICU. He was released 6 days later, without any deficits, to return to his loving wife in a wonderful Cuban community.

To this day, somewhere in American, there is a dead patient walking around, first pronounced by Dr. Carbona and then saved by two Paramedics, two EMTs and a gaggle of firefighters.

…………..

It was not uncommon in the early days for Ambulances to park at street corners, as most systems didn't have substations.

In our town, the drive-in was a great place to "stage."

We got to watch whatever movies there were, for free, and it was easy egress in case of a call.

At some point during the evening, the driver leaned his head towards the corner of the driver's seat and dozed off.

At some other point, his partner, laying in the back, had the need to visit nature and exited the unit from the rear to find a tree.

The radio blared.

"Unit 63", he said. The driver startled up and grabbed the microphone.

"At the drive in", he reported.

"Start towards downtown for a call."

"10-4," he replied. He turned the key, gunned the engine, and they were off to a call.

Well, almost *they.*

As the Ambulance zoomed past the tree, the partner, still taking nature on a walk, stared as his Ambulance pulled out of the drive in and turning it's red lights on, blared down to the interstate entrance and up on the highway.

Great, the partner thought.

Having no cell phones in the day, he went to a payphone and called dispatch.

"2200 hours Ambulance service," the dispatcher answered (you have to remember that, in those day, the only way we knew what time the recorder was recording was to state the time at the beginning of the conversation).

"Hey, this is Phil on 63. My Ambulance just left the drive-in without me and I don't think he knew I'm not there."

That didn't make sense. They both sat next to each other. How could he not tell?

"What are you saying?" dispatch asked.

"He thinks I'm in the back," he said. It started to become clear to dispatch.

It also started to become obvious to the driver.

As the Ambulance careened down the highway, lights and sirens blaring, the driver leaned back towards the rear window and yelled for his partner to get up and that they had a call.

No movement.

He looked in the rear view mirror and realized his partner was not in the Ambulance.

He shut down his lights and sirens and slowed to a normal speed. *Someone needed to know that I was missing my partner,* he thought.

The radio crackled again.

"Unit 63 to dispatch," he announced.

"Go ahead 63", the dispatcher announced. He had already taken the time to call a unit that actually *had* two people to respond to the call, essentially cancelling the call from the 1-man unit. He hadn't called them yet, as he wanted to see how this played out.

"We have to cancel ourselves on this call," he said.

Never in the history of the company had an Ambulance cancelled themselves. Dispatch was totally responsible for that process.

Now, several Managers had gathered in dispatch, hearing the predicament.

"You can't cancel yourself," the dispatcher answered. "Continue on the call."

"We *must* cancel," he repeated. "We are missing a piece of *equipment.*"

Now, everyone was on board with messing with this unit to the wall.

"Let me know what piece of equipment you're missing and I'll have a Supervisor bring it to you," dispatch answered.

The driver was now getting worried. Where was his partner? What if he fell out onto the highway and had been killed by a truck? What if he was kidnapped?

"My Supervisor doesn't *have* this kind of equipment," he answered, trying not to let anyone know he had lost ½ of his crew.

Now, the laughing in the background was too telling.

"Unit 63," he chuckled. "Go back to the drive in and pick up your partner."

The radio was silent.

As the driver got off of the interstate to return to the drive in, he wondered how dispatch would have known where he left him.

As he pulled into the drive in, he spotted his partner, a large soft drink in his hand, leaning against the wall of the concession stand.

And, so it goes.

This is the story of the Ambulance crew member who found out his wife had a great paying job.

He just didn't know what the job was, or where.

The Odd Place was the bar where women danced, almost naked, in cages.

I truly never thought any of these places existed, except in television. Being someone who didn't drink, I knew most bars to be somewhat dark and dismal.

Jerry Matthews and Mac Olbright were two of the four nighttime crews. Typical night guys, they worked in the darkness and slept during the day.

Jerry was single, about 30, somewhat heavy but very active in the company softball team. He loved what he did and figured he had a few more years to pay off some bills and then move on to nursing.

Mac was younger, still very star struck by the whole Ambulance thing. He was married for about a year to a wonderful, energetic and hard-working young lady. She had just gotten a job paying *great* money, at least from what Mac could tell, and that certainly didn't hurt as they were like most young couples. They weren't struggling but they weren't swimming in money either.

On this night, Jerry and Mac were parked on the corner of I-275 and Dale Mabry highway, as they were on most nights. It seemed quiet, although it was only midnight.

Suddenly, the radio came to life.

"Unit 70," dispatched called.

"Dale *Mayberry* and I-275" Jerry answered. They enjoyed mispronouncing the highway.

"Respond to the Odd Place, report of a fall," the radio droned.

"Copy, we're right across the street, put us 97," the radio lingo for being on scene.

Jerry drove the Ambulance across the street and parked to the side of the building. You never want to park right in front of the door where the drunks exited. More often than not, you were guaranteed to have one or two customers sleeping inside when you returned. They always mistook your Ambulance for the local drunk bus.

Mac jumped out and grabbed his "jump kit," appropriately named as you grabbed it and "jumped" to the call. It contained the basics involving first aid and airway.

As Mac entered the door, he scanned the floor, assuming he would find the patient at that level. Quickly, he saw the injured man, lying to the side, a victim of a hard floor and a harder bar stool. A small amount of blood was dripping off of his ear onto the floor. The music was deafening.

He kneeled down near the man and helped him prop himself up against the bar and started to assess the injury and his vitals.

Mac never looked up but had that sixth sense that his partner was standing right next to him.

"GAUZE!" he screamed out over the music. A good medic needed only to give the first word of a path of treatment and the other part of the team would know what followed next.

Placing the bandage on the cut of the patient, he held his hand out, expecting a roll of gauze to secure it.

His hand remained empty.

"HEY, HOW ABOUT SOME ROLLER GAUZE?" he screamed again, wishing they would just stop the music for a minute.

Failing to have any reaction, he finally looked up at Jerry and saw him staring off towards the back of the room.

'WHAT THE HELL ARE YOU LOOKING AT?" Mac yelled again. "HAVEN'T YOU SEEN A NAKED LADY BEFORE?"

Mac thought he heard the word, "wife" come from Jerry's mouth but he couldn't be sure because of the noise. Besides, Jerry wasn't married and, as for Mac's wife, she certainly didn't have anything to do with this call.

Quickly, Jerry looked down at Mac, kneeling next to the patient, who had a half-ticked and half questionable facial expression. Realizing Mac couldn't hear him, Jerry raised his voice and repeated, this time with more volume.

"YOUR WIFE!" he yelled now.

Mac looked up.

While kneeling next to his patient who had fallen and bumped his head, Mac's wife was dancing, naked, in a cage.

It was, as if time froze for both men.

Jerry realized that his partner, now looking pretty dismal and in disbelief, saw her dancing. He grabbed a role of gauze and knelt down next to Mac. He leaned over and, as privately as he could, yelled in his ear.

"I'LL TAKE IT FROM HERE," Jerry said. "YOU GO GET THE STRETCHER."

Mac didn't move. He looked like he wasn't breathing. Jerry was sure he wasn't blinking. After several more prods from Jerry, Mac got up and walked towards the cage.

Jerry couldn't stop him.

As he got closer and closer, I watched as Nancy, his relatively new wife of 1 year, continued to dance, oblivious that her husband was in the audience.

Finally, you could see in her eyes that she recognized him. At the moment their eyes met, the rhythm that drove her body all but stopped. She stared at her husband and, it appeared, became terribly embarrassed.

He stood, she stood. The music was *terribly* blaring and almost deafening. She started to cry in the cage. Mac turned and went out the door.

As Nancy exited the cage and went back stage, Mac returned with the stretcher. By that time, the patient had told Jerry that he didn't want to go and would get a cab home. Mac took the stretcher back and returned with the clipboard, where Jerry had the patient sign a release and refusal of transport.

They both exited the bar. As the door closed, the loudness of the music faded and Jerry's head stopped hurting.

"What are you doing here?" Nancy said, standing beside our unit, now fully clothed,

"WHAT AM I DOING HERE?" Mac screamed. "WHAT THE HELL ARE **YOU** DOING HERE?"

"I told you that I had gotten a job," she told him, as if that was the answer he was looking for.

Mac didn't answer. He climbed into the driver's seat and yelled for Jerry to get in.

Jerry looked into Nancy's eyes. There was hurt, embarrassment, surprise – all wrapped up in a pile of big tears.

"ARE YOU COMING OR NOT?" Mac yelled at his partner. Jerry climbed into the passenger seat.

"Are you ok to drive?" Jerry asked.

Mac suddenly had one of the calmest voices Jerry had heard from him in some time.

"Why wouldn't I be?" He asked as if he was asking for the time.

Before Jerry could explain that the fact that he found his wife dancing naked at the Odd Place may hinder his safe driving habits, they peeled out onto Dale Mabry Highway. Mac picked up the microphone.

"Dispatch, unit 70 is 10-7," using the radio code for out of service. "We need to come into base."

Dispatch acknowledged and, with that, an Ambulance with a car following behind, travelled quickly to headquarters. They both screeched into the parking lot.

"Mac," Jerry tried to reason. "It's just a job. It pays good. What's the big deal?"

Jerry didn't know why he said that. He was simply trying to stop a potential divorce from occurring – at least, while on his shift.

Eventually, Mac went home (without his wife) and Jerry got another partner for the evening.

The final thought on this? Well, there are many, but Jerry learned a valuable lesson. Never look at the dancer's faces. You don't know who you'll meet.

Customer Service

You might think, by the title, that this is going to be another chapter about the excellence in customer service we should be giving to our patients.

You would be wrong.

Instead, I'm going to tell you a story.

I am sitting in a large, rather well-known hotel chain's restaurant, attempting to get breakfast.

I have traveled to this city of 2 million to attend a meeting and had the morning to myself. I was greeted to sit at a table in the central section of the establishment, given a menu – and forgotten.

For the next 25 minutes, I will sit and watch what was wrong with customer service.

Seated in the same serving area were three parties. One table had four men in business suits. The other two had couples. I was alone. I don't think that made any difference, but it was apparent that I was invisible to the staff.

While waitress after waitress flittered around the three tables, assisted by no more than two others, I sat without water, without coffee and without an order.

This goes on for 25 minutes.

Mind you, most of the waiting staff and their assistants walked by my table when they had nothing to do at that moment, hands empty. They never looked my way, never asked why my table was without water – if I was breathing.

Finally, a waitress I had never seen in this area and told me she'd be there in a minute.

Since it had been 25, what was another minute?

That time period lasted 5 minutes. She arrived at my table. No apology. No note that she even acknowledged my inconvenience at waiting a half an hour for someone to discover that I was hungry.

The food was fine. When I was finished, it took another 15 minutes to get a check.

As I wrote my displeasure on the check, my waitress arrived and scolded me for writing on the check. "I'll have to get another one for the cashier" and wandered off to get the paperwork straight. She never asked **what** I was writing.

As I exited the restaurant and went over to the Manager, I realized that this issue was not solely a property of a restaurant or a hotel.

Customer Service in EMS is focused on the patient, as it should be, however, sometimes (actually, probably more than we want to admit), as Managers, we forget that the internal customers are also in need of service. The internal customers range from police Officers, to Hospital staff, to other EMS providers, first responders and, yes, even your own people.

Instead, we flit around them doing "important things" and never acknowledge their presence, their hard work or their commitment to the mission.

When we do finally realize they are there, we don't mention the "inconvenience" they may have suffered (sorry you didn't get off on time) or the sacrifices they make every day to do the right thing (so, how are you doing after that baby drowning?).

I made myself a promise when I became a Supervisor that I would never forget that. I would try to acknowledge everyone I came in contact with and make sure they knew, that I knew, how important they were in the mission and in my life.

It is not only the customer we should focus on, our co-workers. We often times forget about the "other" customers – the ones at home, that family who loves us deeply and wants us to come home safe every night.

If you are one of these co-workers, one who works a shift on an EMS, fire or law enforcement shift, please remember what your family wants most from you. It isn't fancy clothes or a car or even a bigger TV. They want something that can't be bought with overtime, can't be measured and can't be "handed-off" to someone else.

It's our time. They would like us to acknowledge our love for them by simply being with them.

It could be sitting at home watching a favorite TV show (yes, that is quality time, no matter what the counselors say) to playing a board game to simply listening to what kind of day they had.

Sound boring? Not at all. They are the reason we do everything we do, aren't they? Whether it is a husband, wife, boyfriend, girlfriend, roommate or whomever you share your life with – make sure you are making the same commitment to them as you do to the strangers you meet every day.

A friend of mine gave me a great idea. I can't believe after doing this for 39 years, I hadn't thought of it. Another Manager had told me that he writes to all of the families, particularly the children, whose member is working during the Christmas holidays. He apologizes to them for their absence during the holiday but lets them know how many lives they are touching during these times and, regardless of the need for them to work, hopes their Christmas is a bright one.

Isn't that a *great* idea? Thanks, Chris. I'm going to start doing that for our employees this Christmas.

One final thought that we all need to keep in mind. The customers you greet and swear to give the best service to – the truth is that you will probably not see them again. That doesn't mean we shouldn't give them 100% of our time and energy and make sure that their care is the best we can give, but usually, they are a one-time customer.

What about your external customers (family) at home? You see them every day – unless you drop the ball on that end of customer service. Should you fail at that customer service survey, believe me, one day, they'll be gone. At first, you won't know why - but when it does hit you, that you may have not given them the best customer service you could (100%), it will hurt you like nothing has ever hurt.

I am blessed enough to have a family that, early on in my life, I realized the importance of external customer service. I have often asked my wife (reflecting) if I had ever missed many of Robert's games or school activities. She smiles and tells me not to worry and that it seemed like I was there almost all the time. That makes me feel better, however, I still watch today, even with my son grown and out of the house, when I think I am shying away from telling my family how much I love them and giving them time with all of us to talk, watch TV, go to a movie or scuba dive.

It doesn't matter *what* you do with them as much as the *time* you spend with them. Shorten that, cheat that time, and one day, for a reason you will often not be able to find, they will be gone. All for an issue, more time, that you could have fixed easily.

And that would be a tragedy of epic proportions.

Lightning

The sound that Jerry heard was quick, very loud and powerful. The light from the storm was so immense and, yet, blinding. He briefly lost consciousness and when he came to, was twenty to thirty feet away from where he had been – he thought. He really didn't know and couldn't remember.

Jerry and his friend had been collecting from Jerry's newspaper route and had been doing really well in this retirement trailer community. In some communities, people were either not home or simply didn't answer. This Saturday, most were home and happily gave them what was owed. It was a good day.

Suddenly, a strong thunderstorm rumbled over them as the rain started to pour. They both ran for cover under two large oak trees next to the houses.

Soaked, they both stopped under separate trees, no more than 50 feet from one another. Both looked at one another, laughing at each other being wet as fish. They stopped laughing and smiled at each other as Chad, the 14 year old, leaned against his tree and started to count his money. Jerry, 15, had decided to take a leak against his tree. No one appeared to be looking.

Then, it happened.

Jerry found himself on the ground, in almost a seizure like activity. He didn't understand what was happening but he knew he was in pain.

How did I get here? Where am I? What happened?

With the rain still pouring in buckets, the sirens approached and he heard voices. He looked up to see someone in a uniform.

"I'm Don, what happened?" the man in the uniform said.

Jerry couldn't answer. It was as if he was somewhat paralyzed. In some ways, he didn't understand what the man was saying – but he did. It was very strange.

"Over here," he heard a voice.

After checking him out for wounds, bleeding or other injuries. Finding none, the man in the uniform told the child on the ground, "I'll be back in a minute,"

Don ran over to another man in uniform who was huddling over…..well, over something. Jerry didn't recognize what it was – or who it was. He was still confused as to what he was doing outside in the rain and on the ground.

Both men returned to where Jerry was at and quickly started to put him on a board, strapping his body down and making him comfortable.

What happened, Jerry thought? *Why can't I stop shaking?*

Don and his partner moved the teen to the stretcher, now also soaked, and to the Ambulance. This was one of the worst storms they had ever seen and the lightning was wicked. As they loaded the boy, a large bolt of lightning hit the sky, followed by loud thunder. Both Paramedics jerked, huddled down towards the ground while pushing the stretcher into the unit, closing the door behind them.

....

That had happened sometime around 1984 and I hadn't thought of it in years, but as I stood on the porch of my home in 2014, on fire from a direct hit of lightning, I remembered the power we had been dealing with years ago.

My wife had been in our house with the power out, talking about the day's events. It was unusual that the power would be out, but not totally since there was a severe thunderstorm going on outside.

Suddenly, I realized that I could no longer hear my wife speaking to me. It was as if someone had hit me hard on the head with something and stunned me. I looked over to see why she had stopped talking and noticed that her lips were still moving as if she was trying to tell me something.

I then remembered – *what was that loud noise?*

About 15 seconds after the initial shock, my hearing returned and Barbara was yelling at me that the house was on fire.

Always the professional, I told her it wasn't and to calm down.

"It hit a tree near us, not the house," I said confidently.

I also noticed that Lillie, our Lab, was trying to crawl up my pants leg. She looked very scared.

I got up, walked around to the front of the house and, as I exited, noted that engine 119 from the City Fire Department was running emergency down our street. *Probably a medical call,* I thought.

I walked under the overhang of our front porch to the side and looked up, expecting to see some tree on fire.

There was none – but, there was smoke coming from somewhere in the backyard.

I came inside to find Barbara getting Lilly on her leash and telling me again, in a rather emphatic tone, that our house was on fire.

I calmly dismissed her.

"Dear," I said in my best *everything is going to be ok* voice. "The house is not on fire. We would smell smoke by now." At that moment, I smelled smoke inside our house.

I went out the back door to the porch and looked outside – and what I saw put me in panic mode.

On the 2nd floor, midway between the roofline and a window, was a hole the size of my first – maybe bigger – and flames were shooting out of it.

Barbara and I had a code word we had decided on years ago that, if either one of us were to tell the other that word, that person was to do whatever the code-giver said, quickly and without question.

As I came back into the house we both looked at one another and said the code word to each other at the same time.

"Get Lilly and get out of the house, get into the car and pull it back onto the street away from the house", I yelled, trying to remain calm.

I picked up the phone and called 911. I told them what was happening and confirmed for them that everyone was getting out of the house.

As I exited, there was a fire truck 50 feet down the street just sitting there. I assumed they were looking for us.

As I told the 911 dispatcher that they were there and I was hanging up, I ran out and flagged the fire truck to come closer. I recognized most of the guys on the truck as members of the St. Amie Fire Department, a local Public Safety fire service. We were in the city but both departments worked well together in an automatic aid mode.

I really didn't care as long as they had water and hoses.

"Hey, Chief," the new Captain said through the side window.

"This way guys…..343…..lightning," I said, pushing half words out, sounding as stupid as anyone who's house had been hit by lightning.

"Oh," He said a little surprised. "Your house, too? Well, it's on the screen and they are sending someone. They'll be here in a minute. We're on the way to a transformer fire."

Now, for the record, I want to state that I love my firefighters. Whether they are city, county, Public Safety, whatever, they are some of the bravest folks I know.

But, now, with my house on fire and a fire truck directly in front of it, he was telling me that they were busy with a *transformer* (which I was pretty sure no one lived in) and that someone would be with me in a moment.

I tried to remain calm.

Grabbing the side of the fire truck window, I yelled, "My *HOUSE* is on fire!"

He stopped for a moment, looked at the screen, looked back at my house, looked at me and made, in my opinion, one of the greatest field command decisions I have ever heard (since it was my house, why wouldn't it be?).

"Guys, grab that hydrant there and lay a line," he commanded, pointing to the corner. They pulled around enough to wrap a house to the hydrant, charged the line to the truck and fell into line to enter my house.

Within minutes, a full contingent of fire departments and command vehicles were on site. The fire had been extinguished with minimal damage.

………………..

I remembered how, back whenever, we had started a more thorough physical on the older boy, it became obvious what had taken place. Chad, the younger of the two, had been killed by lightning that hit the tree he was leaning against. Electricity, wanting to find ground, did so by entering his left shoulder and traveling down through his body and out of both of his feet, blowing the soles of both shoes clean off. Both of his feet were still smoking and were burning hot to the touch. His lifeless body lay 20 feet from the tree he had been leaning against.

The younger boy in the Ambulance had been urinating onto the next tree and, probably through a flash of lightning (not a direct hit), had the strike go through the urine stream and – yes, into his body through *that* organ and out both of his feet, singeing his shoes but not blowing the soles out.

As we stripped him of his clothes, looking for any burns or other injuries, we wrapped him in a warm blanket, we placed oxygen on him and within a minute, he started to make more sense. A sheriff department deputy arrived and my partner stepped out to tell him of the dead child and our patient.

"What happened?" he asked again.

"I think you may have been struck by lightning," I said calmly. "Do you have any pain?"

"It really hurt at first – all over – but not much now," he said. "I was under the tree waiting for the rain to stop."

"Do you remember what you were doing before all of this?" I asked.

....

Our house was safe, without power, but no longer on fire. As the firefighters picked up their equipment to leave, I was pulled aside by the battalion Chief.

"Chief, we're going to leave the power off at the box," he said. "The power company will be by later and will pull the meter so that it can't be turned on until you get an electrician to check it all out."

By now, the local Chaplain, Gayle, was there and she was such a comfort. Neighbors came out and offered a place to stay, storage for our food, anything we needed. While it was a scary event, it was also great to see America at its finest.

....

My mind flashed back to the boys' first words after we started his transport.

"I have a paper route," he kept repeating. "Where's Chad?"

My partner had stepped back into the rear of the Ambulance as the questions were asked. We looked at one another.

"Was he with you?" I asked.

"Yeah – he was helping me. Where is he?" He now asked a little more excited.

Of all of the things they teach you in Paramedic school, telling people that their parents, spouses, brothers or sisters, grandparents or just simply, your best buddy – was dead, was not one of them. Later in my career, I would learn the "art" of doing that – but had not at the time of this call.

As I continued to initiate treatment, my partner spoke up.

"He's back where we picked you up with the deputy," he told him. I think he probably knew what had happened but, for the moment, that answer satisfied him.

"So, you were under the tree," I asked again.

"Yeah, I was collecting for my paper route," he repeated.

"Didn't you see the lightning storm?" I asked.

"Sure," he answered. Then, he asked a question, as if he knew how he had ended up on my stretcher.

"Where did it touch me?"

Lightning. He probably didn't "see" it, but he certainly felt it.

Actually, both my partner and I were curious ourselves.

"What was the last thing you remember?" I asked.

"I was under the tree," he repeated. "I was going to the bathroom."

It was, at the exact moment, that all of us got it.

Jerry lifted up the sheet and looked down towards his groin.

"Am I going to be ok?" he asked. I knew what he was asking and understood his fear.

"There aren't any burns or anything," I said. "I think you're going to be ok."

Jerry sighed a relief sound. The IV needle I was starting returned a flash of blood and I hooked up the IV to run at a moderate rate, the protocol at the time for electrical burns.

As I was taping it down, the young child's face took the look of stone again and he looked back up at me.

"Chad's dead, isn't he?" he asked.

I wasn't sure, as I had not seen the patient up close. I looked over at my partner. He slightly nodded his head.

"I think so," I told him.

As we drove away, with lights and sirens blaring, Jerry and I both cried for his friend, someone who was just helping him out with his paper route.

So, on a summer's day, two young teenagers were struck by lightning. In one instant of a second, one was dead and the other alive.

. . . .

On that night in 2014, The night of the lightning strike on our house, as my wife and I cuddled on the king bed at the local motel, Lilly, not used to being in the bedroom, looked at me with a forlorn face. She pawed at the bed.

"Come on," I said and she immediately, as if on cue, jumped up and cuddled into me.

There I was, squeezed between the two females in my life. We were healthy, we were alive. That's all that mattered.

Some are not always that blessed.

1977

"Don," Lee shouted. "How are we going to talk on this portable?"

I looked inside our new unit to see a charging box, bungee-chord around it, attaching it to the wall of the inside, wires, bare and running from the box to somewhere under the cabinet.

"We'll wing it, I guess," I said and smiled.

Lee looked mad, not at me, but at the situation we were in. One of the largest Ambulance services were about to start a Paramedic service in one of largest counties in Florida. We were trying to do it right, but like so many times, the small things weren't covered, so now, we were talking into a glued box with bare wires.

Day one of the Hillsdale Ambulance System starts. There are 14 new box-styled (we called them Type I's or modular) Ambulances stand on the line, ready to be deployed. People meet up in the training room, as others mill about outside, getting equipment ready. We have been waiting for this day since the first day of Paramedic class. Effective today, Paramedics will be in the unincorporated area of the county. We were excited, scared….excited.

"Good morning everyone," I heard a voice. That was Mr. McGovern.

"This morning is historic," he stated. "We have been waiting for years to get this started and, this morning, Paramedics will spread across the county to give our patients the best care possible."

He paused, as if he was thinking of something.

I looked around at the crowd. Yesterday, we were all Basic Life Support providers and, this morning, we were about to depart on an exciting path of Paramedicine.

…………..

It had been nine months since I have seen the sun.

Or, so it seems.

Paramedic class started in August with 21 of us, hand-picked by the Medical Director himself and approved to attend the first Paramedic course in our County.

It was funded through a grant program, so there was no cost to us. There were no books for the course, except that big federal DOT manual. The instructor, Dick and Penny, would ask that we buy an EKG book written by a Doctor named Johnson.

Dr. Dale Johnson was a local plastic surgeon in town. The story goes that one day, while in one of the local Hospitals watching a doc read an EKG, he asked him to explain to him how to read one. He had a small course in school, of course, but since he knew he was going to be a plastic surgeon, he didn't worry about it too much.

After about 20 minutes, Johnson exclaimed, "Well, hell, that's pretty easy. Someone should write a book about that."

And he did. The book remains a standard for the simple interpretation of EKGs.

However, with that exception, everything was done on overheads, copied paper and the chalk board. They explained, showed us, explained some more and, of course, we had Hospital time.

The interview process seemed pretty hard. Questions, mostly about your personal life; Did your wife know about the grueling 24/48 shift, where you spent 24 on the road, 18 hours in the Hospital and 12 hours in class? What does your family think about you getting into this school? Do you like this job?

It seemed to me that there were no medical questions, the ones I had studied for since I got my letter for the interview. They said 60 people were interviewing and only 21 would be accepted. I had studied everything in EMT I could study.

As I was rethinking my knowledge, I realized they had asked one last question.

"What?" I asked.

"We said we appreciated you coming in to interview. One last question – do you know what Ecchymosis is?"

My mind froze.

Of course, I knew what that was – but I was so nervous, my palms were sweating so sweaty, my mind swirling – I had forgotten.

"My apologies," I stated. "I've been so nervous about this interview, my mind has drawn a blank. I've heard of it before, I just can't put my fingers on it."

The Cardiologist on the board tried to give me some hints, "Bruising behind the ears, around the eyes…."

I remained stoic.

"I'm sorry," I repeated. *How pathetic*, I thought. "I just really want to get into this class and have just drawn a blank. It's my nerves, I guess."

They thanked me and let me exit. I knew my goose was cooked.

Later, I heard that another candidate had been asked a different question ("What is Moribund?" – Man, I wish they had asked me THAT one – I KNEW that one). When he also panicked and forgot what it was, he went on a 10 minute diatribe on some mess that had nothing to do with anything. He later told some that he thought he could "bullshit" his way through it.

The following day, the list came out – and I was on it! I couldn't believe after messing up the question, I had been accepted!

The instructor told me later on that not knowing the question, and being *honest* about it, made the difference. The guy who blew his way through fantasyland was NOT accepted. He was mad, but he got over it.

…………..

"You should have your assigned station in a packet in your unit," he continued. "If it is a fire station, they know you are coming this morning. Remember; you are in their house. I expect everyone to be on their best behavior. If you are going to a Hospital, they are also waiting for you and will show you where your rooms are at."

Again, he paused. "For those going to the Midget Motel…."

A few of us chuckled at that, a few whistled. We don't know why to this day we did it - it was just the idea that the powerful Ambulance service, giving extremely great care was going to be stationed at the Midget Motel. Then, the reality set in. Some fire departments didn't *want* us there. They had a good thing going, a few fires every week but, other than that, very quiet. They knew how busy we were and how we would upset the natural order.

Mr. McGovern continued. "Well, they'll give you the key when you get there."

"Good luck and let's make us all proud."

....

I had not been in a real school in five years. I knew it would be hard, but really, I had no idea how hard it would be. I soon found out that I had signed up for mega-school, mixed in with Hospital and clinical time, ride along time and, in between all of that, our regular work. Family came in second when it came to Paramedic school. They had to be in on it; otherwise, you would certainly fail.

They told us at the beginning, any idea of a vacation, time off, moving, job changes, pregnancy (I am not sure how they could control that), and divorces – anything that would disrupt your life would most likely put you in a position of not passing the course. The families understood. We understood. It was what we signed up for.

Over the next nine months, we learned the short course on cardiology, the physiology of the body, its organs, common diseases and injuries found by Paramedics and what to do for them. We learned about different medications, ones the patient had and ones we would give them. We learned algebra (or re-learned it, I suppose) to help us with the drug calculations and complications of the medications we were giving.

We learned how to interpret EKG's, the extrication equipment, the proper way to diagnose difficult diseases and patient care in general.

We went to work on a 24 hour unit, got off shift to drive to the Hospital and do 12 to 14 hour rotations and the next day, classroom from 8:30 to 3 PM.

When we weren't doing all of that, we were doing ride-a-longs and studying. Studying and sleeping.

No – that wasn't correct.

Sleep was optional.

As we gathered our equipment, Lee and I looked at each other and he smiled. Lee was not one to smile much, not that he wasn't a happy person – but he didn't show much of his feelings. He was 100% professional with his patients and knew that many of them would depend upon his expertise in order to live. I had really enjoyed having Lee as my field instructor. He had taught me a great deal about the business and had shown me many medical things I think I would have missed had he not stopped me from what I was doing and said, "Come on upstairs for a minute. I want to show you something." We would wander up to a gallery where they were setting a femur or doing some procedure. He would walk through what they were doing and why it was so important that we did this or that. It made the connection about what we were doing meaningful.

The 14 Ambulances pulled out of the front of the old Funeral Home/headquarters and headed to our stations. On board were 28 new Paramedics, never before being in charge of their own Paramedic truck, counting and re-counting in their heads, the long list of medications they had, where everything was at, what they would carry into the house first.

It had begun.

The Union

I am probably going to make some of my closest friends mad with this chapter, and for that, I apologize.

For those who I do not know, I make no apologies.

I am a Paramedic of 40 years, working in some tremendous organizations and, yes, at one point, a union member.

My union education started in 1977 when the Communications Workers of America (CWA) somehow asked us to join their union. At that time, I didn't understand how a union was formed (a formal letter or petition must be filed with the National Labor Relations Board) or why we needed one, but there they were, telling us our lives would be better than they were now. Who was I to argue?

So, I went to the meeting that explained everything. Several of my co-workers got up and told me what a great thing this would be, to have a professional union to make sure we didn't get "screwed."

I was all in, although I hadn't been "screwed" by anyone in the department, but it sure sounded like we were going to be, so – well, I was in!

That was, until they mentioned that it was only going to cost $12 a pay period.

Cost us? What did they think I was made of – money? They told me, don't worry, we'll get that money back in raises. Raises? I was born at night, but it wasn't last night. We were working, at that time, for a County Government. Raises were few and far between and I didn't know of anyone working for government who got one.

"How were these raises going to come about," I asked?

"You'll have to join to find out," they said.

I declined.

That was where *the voice of the union* started. Everywhere I was, there was someone who had joined, who told me how great the union was. They assured me that it was ok if I didn't want to join right away. I could join later after I had seen the wonderful work they had done to improve our "work environment."

You have to remember that, at the time, we were working out of an old Funeral Home. My boss's office was in a viewing room and we ate in the "prep" room (talk about losing an appetite). We also had stations in several locations across the county, including a hotel (Gibsonton Hotel was my favorite) as well as an old dilapidated house in Plant City. The "working environment" certainly could stand some improvements.

I didn't see, however, how the union was going to do that. Bill, the newly elected President of the union, was a great carpenter but I didn't see him helping the County improve its facilities.

So, I watched and waited – and was both right and wrong.

Over the next four years, they did improve. We built a new headquarters station, complete with a state-of-the-art dispatch center. We teamed up with local fire stations to get into their facilities. We stationed two units at local Hospitals and had nice rooms in which to live there.

The problem was that all of those things were brought about by management. The union had nothing to do with it.

And, yet, *the voice* continued to talk to me.

Yes, the voice told me, *"but they wouldn't have done it if it weren't for the "threat" that the union brought with them."*

What threat was that, I thought? A strike? That was against the law and in the contract they eventually signed with the CWA. Without that threat, all they had was the threat of…..what? I pictured EMTs standing on the corner, carrying signs and yelling unpopular things and basically looking pitiful.

$12 a pay period? I didn't see the value.

The voice continued to talk to me, in various forms, at all times of the day and night while at work and off duty.

"What happens if you get into trouble? Who will represent you?"

"What happens if you get fired? Who will push for your reinstatement?"

In my head, I thought it was doubtful that I would get into trouble or be fired because I didn't do things wrong.

"That doesn't matter," the voice would tell me. *"They're out to fire those they don't like"*.

The more they talked to me, the sillier it sounded. Heck, we couldn't even strike.

So, I did not join.

Over the next few years, the County employees who were unionized received whatever COLA was allowed non-union workers. Any benefit that the union received, non-union also received. I didn't see any benefit.

….until one day when I saw a possible value.

We had been on 24 on/48 off shifts for quite some time. In an attempt to hold down the overtime costs, the department decided to put the entire department on a 12 on, 12 off, four day work week. It sounded reasonable. The 24 hour shift was somewhat long and, even though it would appear we got some down time, there were days you were on the road for an entire 24 hour shift. I will admit that in my 23 hour, I was probably not on my best game. When that involves giving medications in an IV, it can be rather scary.

So, we all went to the 12 on and 12 off shift. Being someone who had been there since the beginning, I opted for the night shift. Becky, my partner, rode with me. We did that for almost one year and, after about six months, it was not the restful shift we all thought it would be.

Unfortunately, the powers that be would not change the shift. The *voice* spoke.

Join us. We'll get your 24 hour shift back for you.

Suddenly, I realized that there was a value to this organization. I didn't have the $12 to spare, but told Barb that we would simply have to do this to make my life at work better.

I joined. I was now a brother.

Negotiations started and although we were not involved with them, we heard from "Ken" the union steward, how difficult management was being but that they were *holding their feel to the fire* and the new contract was coming that we would all like.

A day arrived that an announcement was made that a tentative agreement with management was reached and that we would be voting on the new contract the following Friday. All of us were very excited, slapping Ken on the back and thinking that maybe the *voice* was right after all. We *needed* the union!

Friday came and a small table was set up in the deployment room. Becky and I walked up, presented our ID's and were given a ballot.

Vote to approve the contract and sign the voice said.

"Where's the contract?" we asked.

The voice stopped what he was doing and looked at us as if we had asked a sacrilegious question. *There's one copy on the desk you can read if you want, but basically, we go back to 24/48.*

Ok, I thought. That's good. The contract looked awfully thick, though. What else could be in it?

"Do you mind if I read through it?" I asked.

The voice sighed. *"Sure."*

Becky and I took it to the corner (you would have thought for the money we were paying that they would have given all of us our own copy) and started to read.

"….EMS crews will work a 24/48 hour schedule as deemed by this contract…"

 The next paragraph had to do with pay.

…"crews will be paid 16 hours out of the 24, with 8 hour of unpaid sleep time….."

Unpaid sleep time? Were we LOSING money in order to get our 24 hour shift back?

I asked the *voice* to explain this.

The *voice* looked up at me as if I was stupid. *You have to start somewhere when you negotiate.*

"So," I asked. "You started with my salary and reduced it, thinking I would be ok with that?"

The voice had no answer.

Several of my co-workers around me were like sheep, nodding their heads to the happy notification that we were going back to 24 hour shifts.

I tried to talk sense into many. Most would have none of it.

The final vote? 142 in favor, four against (Becky and I got two more who didn't want to lose pay). The contract passed.

For my $12 a pay period, I learned that I could have an effect on both my schedule and my salary. One was what I had requested and the other – well, I was down almost $3,000 a year (actually $3,312 if you counted my wasted union dues).

So ends my first lesson in a $12 per pay period union political world. Over the next several years, I also noted that when someone did get in trouble, the Union was *almost always* there to fight for them. It did turn out that, even if you were a brother, if they didn't *like* you (or your ethnicity, religion, life style), they would send a representative to a hearing – who would say nothing, even if you paid your $12.

Very democratic.

However, is other cases, when someone did the dumbest thing they could do (sometimes to a patient), they were there to make excuses for the employee and stand with them, no matter how bone-headed they were.

It didn't matter – a union member was NEVER wrong (unless your race, religion, sex or lifestyle got in the way).

There was one more exception to that rule; if you were **not liked** by the Union President, regardless of anything else, you found out the term "union" meant physically something disgusting and generally not physically possible.

The shoes of who was President had changed a few times and Rodger was our new President. I watched the double *The President doesn't like you and we don't like what you do in your private life* scenario when he decided he didn't like one of the best Paramedics we had in the agency (evidently, this employee wasn't dating enough women for his taste) and, one day, told him that the union was not going to represent him in his grievance matter.

Never mind that the employee hadn't done anything wrong – if you were liked, you were good. If not, go to hell.

Therein lies the 2nd lesson of union politics. You shall be *one of the boys* only if they *say* you're one. $12 means nothing.

But, that was not the last of the lessons in Unions I had to endure.

My first job as an EMS Director involved a County who had just filed a request to unionize with another large Public Safety agency which will remain nameless but whose motto is, "There is nothing that can't be solved by adding a big red truck with six more union members."

Now, I was on the other side – the side of management. My boss made no excuses that my first goal was to try to find out what the issues were and to see if I could either talk them out of voting a union in, or at least delay a vote for one year while we fixed whatever the issue was.

I spent a tremendous amount of time asking around and found the one issue to be very simple. When EMS had been transferred from the Sheriff's department to a separate agency under the County, the employees lost some annual leave due to the way it was calculated and spent. It appeared that about 18 hours had to be added to their accounts and all would be well.

I went to the upper management and explained the issue. They saw it, realized that this was a mistake on their part and their plan was fix it by adding the appropriate time to everyone's annual leave account.

You can read about what happened in detail in my chapter *1988* but, let's just say the vote didn't go quite like I thought it would.

And, it was our fault.

However, there was more than what was in that chapter.

Days before the vote, most of the employees had said they were willing to give the County the benefit of the doubt and wait while they fixed this problem. Union dues were $35 a pay period, a much steeper amount than what I remembered.

Then, *the voice* returned – with trays of raw oysters!

Every station we had was visited by a member of the union the night before the vote with a large tray of oysters on ice, letting them know that the union cared about them and there would be more if they voted yes.

And, evidently, that was all it took.

The final vote? Well the union won.

And, the department never excelled at anything again.

My lesson? I should have bought oysters.

EASY OR HARD

Before I started in EMS, I was a private investigator for a hotel chain. As exciting as that sounded, it was just a job – and I saw the ad for dispatcher in the newspaper that would start my career in EMS.

Many told me it sounded like a job that was too hard. It didn't sound like that to me and, besides, so what if it was? I'd just adapt and conquer. I started and realized it <u>was</u> very hard but, with time, I learned the job and, in fact, became quite good at it.

Then, it was on to EMT. Not an easy task since everyone told me that "dispatchers didn't belong in the street." I had to take my class across the Bay in St. Petersburg because my boss told me I would never amount of anything, particularly a good EMT.

That was hard, too, and I soon found that, with that challenge, I started to make straight A's; something that my mother would have been extremely proud of (I was a "C" student in High School). I started to "love" what I was learning and I soon found the "passion" for taking care of patients. I couldn't wait to get to the street.

Then, the hardest part became making the transition. You will have read several parts of that in this book, but I want to talk about it being hard – hard in the fact that I was about to step into "the street," that magical place where the other EMTs went and, for quite some time, I couldn't. I remember the first day of street duty. I worked with Lee (you remember from that chapter). He was so stern, yet calming and assuring. Yet, I was really scared. I didn't think I could do this.

And, then, the first patient – a Cuban speaking older woman who had some belly pain – she couldn't speak English and couldn't tell me much information. I had a set of vitals and my nifty clipboard out, ready to write down what the patient told me about her problem.

What was I doing here? Hard? This was impossible. Yet, with time (and many, many partners and patients), I learned to love it – and have the passion that I had first felt in class.

Over the years, I have had many people ask me why I became a Paramedic. I've told them, for the most part, I never picked the career. The career picked me. While many would talk about the lives saved, I remember hundreds of patients who had nothing more than belly pain or were so weak from old age; they could not walk, but needed to see a Doctor for a minor issue. Those, to me, were the best calls.

These patients were scared to death, having called 911 for what they believed to be the most horrible time in their life. I, the thin (yes, there *was* a day), handsome *(ok, I hear you, cut it out)* Paramedic arrives in time to hold their hand or put my hand on their shoulder, look into their eyes and tell them, "Don't worry Mrs. Strickland, nothing is going to happen while you're with me".

Immediately, her eyes become less scared and she smiles. She tells me about her granddaughter and how she just competed in a dance recital. I ask if she has a picture of her and she quickly reaches over to the nightstand and shows me a small picture of a child.

"Isn't she darling?" she asks. And, with a smile, I make her day.

Believe it or not, *that* is what makes my day. The passion I have for doing the best I can do in the back of a rolling box, whether it's trying to save a life or comforting someone in need of comfort, is something I seem to excel in. Often, when people ask me why I got into EMS, I mention my mother's heart attack when I was a teenager and how helpless I felt.

I am pretty sure that I decided at that moment, as a scared 14 year old with my Mother dying in her bed, that I would help people and train myself so I would never feel that helpless again.

There are many people who tell me, "I couldn't do what you do." My brother makes it more personal. "I'm sure glad there are people like you because I SURE couldn't do that job."

I always tell them that isn't necessarily true.

Everyone does my job every day, in some way or another. Maybe not in the "save the baby from the river" sort of way, but every person has their own "save," in one way or another.

Some truly have that moment of actually saving a life - a friend falls and cuts themselves, a neighbor calls because their child has a fever and they don't know what to do, or maybe it's a total stranger in a restaurant who finds themselves in trouble because they don't feel good.

Are they "saving lives?" That depends on how you look at it. They needed someone and you were there. I bet if you asked them, they would say you did save their life.

Others do my job on a more social level – sometimes saving lives over a period of time – helping a family member addicted to some substance, a friend who is suffering from the death of a family member or a pet ("What's the difference?", some would ask but those who do have never owned a pet), or a friend who simply cannot cope with life – these folks come to us and ask for help.

As you read this, in fact, you probably have pictured the face of that special person in your head and realize – hey! yeah!! I guess I DID save a life! You listened to them as they described the demons in their head, cried with them while they told you of the love they have lost, talked in a loving way of their pet and their antics and listened to them for hours on the phone, not giving any opinion but just being there – a friendly shoulder - until the crisis, whatever it might have been, had passed.

Maybe it wasn't that dramatic. One night, you may have sat with a close friend whose wife had left them after 10 years of marriage – or that special person in your life who is hurt by a word or deed. In any event, you did that – you were a caregiver. You didn't jump into a burning house or do CPR on a child. Believe me, many of us never get that level of true "lifesaving" and, for those of us who do, it is rare, maybe once or twice in a lifetime.

Were we talking about what's hard? Believe me, what you did WAS hard! It wasn't easy doing any of it. There were times, if it was a multi-faceted save (a phone call over many times or a meeting with someone several days in a year) that you probably tried to think of ways to get out of it.

But, you didn't. And, regardless of whether they told you, they – that person who you saved – is grateful for what you did.

Some of you, while you are reading this, may be right in the middle of helping a friend or family member during a life-threatening crisis. One word of advice I would give you is – don't give up. Don't give up on them, on the issue, on the "hook" that you have in their life. They are counting on you.

Is that the hard part? Yeah, I guess it is. I always fall back on a word of advice I got from a TV show (yeah, so it wasn't my long lost uncle but it's still just as good).

"Of course it's hard – it's supposed to be. If it were easy, everyone would do it."

In any event, thanks for being there for whoever it is. Thanks for being that lifesaver, companion, or shoulder to lean on, that person who listens without judgment. You will never know the hundreds that you have helped. But, you did.

It is hard.

1988

"I'd hate for something to happen to your beautiful family."

I hung up the phone.

Over the past few weeks, we have been getting more and more of those kinds of calls. Many were threats, to me and my family, from the union.

I'm not sure if the union knew that their members were doing it – but, then again, it didn't matter.

My goal throughout the entire union negotiations was to not let my family know what those calls were about.

I turned to go towards the family room. Barbara stood in front of me.

"Another one?" She asked. I shook my head.

Barb was a smart woman, probably the smartest I ever met. I have no idea what made her pick me but I know I was lucky.

When I first arrived in Port Englewood, I was excited and amazed. The group of Paramedics and EMTs working there were fabulous. Very focused on patient care and proud of the work they did.

Port Englewood was a small, retired town with about 80,000 people, which increased to around 140,000 during the winter. The influx of "snowbirds" as they were called was seen in the traffic and incidents we responded to.

While the Fire Department was like any other in any other city (dedicated, proud), there was an undertone of unhappiness.

I was asked to a meeting with Ron and the new Fire Chief, hired one week after me, to discuss it.

"They want to form a union," my boss, Ron said. He had been the Fire Chief before being promoted to Public Safety Director. He was over both Fire and EMS.

"Your first mission is to see if you can change their mind," he told me.

"I'm your guy," I said confidently. "I just need to know one thing."

He looked at me, smiled and told me anything I needed was mine.

"Why do they want a union?" I asked.

His smile went away. The Fire Chief remained quiet.

"How the hell do I know?" he groused. "There are some sad-sacks, out of touch, don't-wanna-work-no-more folks who will be unhappy no matter what we do."

I wasn't satisfied.

"With all due respect," I stated, and immediately saw his face turn to a not-smile, close to mad look. "There's always something that is the straw. Has anyone asked them why?"

He told me no, because the petition had already been filed.

For those who don't know how it works, in a non-union setting, personnel must file a petition to vote for whether people want a union at a place of work. There has to be at least 51% of the personnel who sign the petition and it must be presented to the governing agency (in this case, the IRB) in order for a vote to be taken.

90 days after that petition is turned in, a vote takes place. In those 90 days, it is assumed that each side will plead their case as to why it either is or is not needed. There can be no threats of job lost, terminations or other adverse actions in regards to the petition.

"Do you mind if I ask?" I asked. He now seemed absolutely angry.

"No, hell, go ahead and ask your stupid questions," he said. "It won't matter."

The Chief and I left, I with less than a satisfactory feeling that Ron and I both understood the mission at hand.

"Don't you think that makes sense?" I asked the Chief.

"Sure, sure," he said, as if he didn't care either. "He's right though. If they filed, they're going to form a union."

That's the spirit, I thought.

For the next 80 days, I asked everyone in my agency that question. Through some miracle, I got the answer.

Two years earlier, they had transitioned from the local Sheriff department to an EMS system. In that transition, prior to leaving the Sheriff department, they had worked in a system where, if you took 24 hours of annual leave, they were only charged for 16 hours.

The idea was that for at least 8 hours, they slept and shouldn't be charged for annual leave in that period. Only an elected person could do such a thing, however, it was what it was.

When they came to the County, they were told they were to be charged for all hours taken. In their mind, they were losing 20% of their annual leave.

It made sense to me. After working with leading employees on the solution, I contacted my boss and, with HR, everyone agreed that pushing 20% more annual leave into their leave banks would fix that problem.

While that was a simple answer, complications and timing would change history.

While HR was working on that solution, their boss called and mentioned that they had a mandate to put out an employee manual to every employee by June 1st. This was a federal mandate and the date was 4 days before the union vote.

My command staff and the HR Director met in our office to hand out the employee handbooks. She mentioned there were a few "misprints" that we needed to know so we could explain it to the employees.

"Let's take a look on page 6," she stated. "You can see that the figure of 104 hours of annual leave per years was printed wrong. It says 20 but that's supposed to be 104."

All of us looked at her in disbelief.

"So," I stated. "You're going to correct that and get us new books?"

"There's no time," she said. "Just hand them out and explain it to them. Now on page 8…."

"Wait a minute," I demanded. "You can't expect us to hand out a book that, in print, takes away valuable benefits already promised by the County and then in the same breath say it was just a mistake and don't pay any attention to it?"

She stared as us with as bank a stare as I have ever seen.

"Yes," she replied in monotone.

"Can't we wait until after the vote to do this?" I stated. "This will be catastrophic for the vote."

"I'm afraid not," she said. "The feds say we have to do this by Monday or we're in violation."

I was the first one to hear it under someone's breath.....

...."Violation of being stupid...." I knew who had said it, but I didn't want to point them out, mostly because they were so correct.

Trying to steer the now icy-cold stare from our HR Director away from the violator, I raised my voice.

"Don't you know we are trying to get hours ADDED to their bank and you want us to sell this?" I questioned. "I don't know how that's going to happen."

"You simply open your mouth and start talking," she said. Her cold stare now aimed straight at me. "You do know how to do that, don't you?" A bit of sarcasm never hurt when you were trying to save the agency.

"Yes mam," I said. I wasn't before, but I was now – afraid of her.

"As I was saying, on page 8..." and she went on to talk about a total of 8 *misprints* which changed the very basic foundation of benefits within the agency.

When she left, I looked at the command staff.

"Well, don't just stand there," I said, somewhat smiling. "Let's go sell it."

Slowly, everyone got up one at a time and walked out with the confidence of Paramedic whose patient was dying but who didn't want to let them know. The patient knew and you knew and no one wanted to talk about it. I watched their faces as they left. Defeat was the look I was not looking for.

All went out and tried to sell it. With a smile on their face and a song in their heart.

The vote took place that next Thursday with 45 voting for it and 3 voting against. So much for selling.

And, with a twist of timing and stupidity, the EMS union, formed alongside the fire union, was formed and, for the next 5 years, made a mockery of the County. When negotiations weren't going well, they called department heads and threatened them and their family.

As the Contract finally was approved, the union got nothing more for their members than what other County employees got. No pay raises, no higher annual leave, no extra bonuses. They did get a mustache policy and the union held a beer bash twice a year.

From a leader's perspective, a union contract made my job much easier.

"No, I can't let you go on annual leave with three days' notice," I would tell one of the union leaders. "The contract says you have to give me 5 days' notice. Sorry."

"But, Boss," he said. "I've worked here for 15 years – doesn't that county for something?"

"Yes, it does," I stated. "However, I can't violate the contract."

I felt bad that I couldn't do things *the way we used to* but it was a new day. The contract was the contract and as long as I followed it, I knew we were all in compliance.

So, with that said, especially during negotiations, calls were *anonymously* made to my phone (and to others) who didn't support the union. Vial, disgusting, dangerous things were said about what they were going to do to us and our families. I knew the threats were full of water as none of those threatening were man enough to do it face to face, but still, with a 4 year old at home, it concerned us.

One day, County Council got a large 8X10 black and white picture of my son exiting out of my County vehicle at his school. The one I saw had a gun site on his head.

I didn't ask who sent it. It didn't matter. Later, I found out that the Fire Marshall at the time, an avid Photographer, took the picture and developed it in his own lab at his house.

Ahhh…the games the union plays.

Of course, the union leaders said that *they* certainly didn't send such a picture and *they* didn't call my house and threaten to kill me and my family in a suspicious house fire.

Yeah......right.

The way I left the service was rather interesting. I have a chapter about that later in the book.

As I left that service, I followed them for a while. They produced no national honors, no local honors, nothing that would put them up to pace with the best. They did well, taking care of the community and, I guess if you want to just *do the minimum*, that's all that you could ask.

It was too bad that the union was formed, in my opinion. The EMS service, at the time, was up for a National Association of Counties Award. The kybosh was soon put on that as it made one of the entities better than the other and, in union rules that was a no-no. Everyone was the same, no one could be special. It took a lot of the growth and innovation out of the service. It made quite a few employees happy, though, so I guess not all was lost.

Unions can be good and bad. There are many places that need one in order to set the course for the future. However, in most cases, it ends up being a business (the union) bent on making money for the national and giving pittance to the members.

I never understood why anyone would pay someone else to represent them to their boss, especially in a place where you could walk up and talk to the boss directly.

Then, again, I'm no union guy.

The Baby

It was just a garbage can.

Not unlike those cans you see at all of the restaurants and service stations across the land. It was gray, with a rounded top and one of those flip doors you push in when you dispose of whatever you are disposing of.

The call came to us as "nature unknown." In this business, you get quite a bit of that and, after a while, if you aren't checking yourself, you'll get a little complacent. The 30th or 40th "nature unknown" that ends up being a boo-boo on a boo-boo gets your thought process to a "nature nothing going on here" mode, so you may not be as alert or cautious when you enter such situations.

We had not had an unusual amount of those calls however, so we were still somewhat awake and alert to what was happening. The call was to a popular hotel chain, right at the bottom of an overpass to one of the many interstates in Florida.

"Nature unknown." How bad could it be?

The first thing we noticed as we pulled into the parking lot was that it was full of cops. Cars at the office, cars at one of the row of rooms, with a 2nd floor room door open and several in between. We weren't sure where we were going, so we ambled towards the open room.

About half way there, we heard a voice.

"Hey," one of the police Officers said. He was in a suit and, although we had a great relationship with most, if not all of the street cops, this guy must be a Detective. Neither I nor my partner recognized him.

"Over here," was all he said, pointing towards the office.

"Must be a fight," I told Jim. "Why don't you wander up to the room and I'll meander back to the office."

In assault cases, especially for EMS, that was sometimes the best thing you could do. Keep the parties separate while you discuss their injuries and what Hospital they wanted to go to. If everyone was in the same room, the conversation usually started with, "He's a no good &*#$%" followed by someone, usually drunk, lunging towards the other person. From that point on, a good medical history was hard, if not impossible to get.

I got out of the right side (it was Jim's turn to drive) and opened the side door to grab a jump kit and started to walk towards the Detective.

The Detective gave me a strange look but said nothing. I walked the 50 yards or so to meet him in the parking area just before you got to the front of the office.

"Well?" I asked, wondering where the patient was.

"How did you get this call?" he asked.

"Nature unknown," I replied. I know that sounds like an incomplete sentence, but often, vowels and other extra words we would normally use in a conversation were lost in many discussions between Law, Fire and EMS. We all seemed to know the unspoken language of "just the facts, Mam'." Sort of like grunting, only with words.

"Oh," he said without an expression to be seen. "Sorry. He's right here."

With that, he pointed to the gray garbage can, top off, that was standing next to the Detective. Had he not of pointed that out, I would have simply walked by and kept going to the office to find whoever needed my assistance.

I looked at him with that, "what the.." look and took a glimpse in to see one of the most horrible scenes I have ever had in my career.

At this point, I had been a Paramedic for about four years. I knew, at some point, I would see "the horror" as we talked about it, some decapitation, some wound that was unbelievable, some weapon used that would cause a deadly, disgusting, bloody mess.

Instead, I saw garbage.

As I looked closer, in between a discarded paper cup, top still on and straw sticking out, and a brown bag of what appeared to be some kind of bottle in it, was the top of a baby's head.

Yes, I thought, that's what that is – a baby. I reached out and the Detective grabbed my hand.

"Don't touch it," he said. "He's cold. Been dead for at least a few hours."

Not to be outwitted by a cop, I smiled and said, "If you want my official opinion, I have to see if I feel a pulse."

"Ok," he said. "But try not to move anything if you can."

I reached down and, as my fingers touched the top of the baby's head, it was obvious that he was a cold as most of what lay with him. I can't really describe the feeling – cold, not moist, not living, cold. He appeared to be almost standing in the can, feet way down towards the bottom and the baby's little head sitting on the top.

How could anyone do this to a baby?

I continued to move my hand down alongside the baby's head, trying to find a pulse in the neck. I knew finding a baby's carotid was difficult as what they train you to do is find his left nipple and feel alongside of it. I wasn't going to be able to reach that without moving a significant amount of garbage.

My hand reached the baby's nose and mouth and I felt. No, no breathing. He was very, very cold.

I pulled my hand out. My face must have told the Detective what he needed to know.

"Signal 7," he said to another Officer, who had appeared without me even knowing he approached us. That was the radio code for Dead on Arrival, the sign that the ME (Medical Examiner) had to be called.

I always thought it silly that EMTs and Paramedics could not, by law, pronounce anyone dead. If they didn't have a pulse, we did CPR. Of course, there were those serious cases, where they were cold and stiff, or had an injury which was incompatible with life. However, if it appeared that CPR would not work and that they were – well, dead, we had to notify the medical examiner.

In many States, they call them the Coroner and, in those cases, they are elected. They would come to the scene, *only after EMS had arrived and pronounced the patient dead,* which of course, we couldn't do. WE pronounced and the ME or Coroner came to us, but – well, you see the dilemma. So, I guess we did, in every way, pronounce the patient – even if we couldn't – and the ME or corner confirmed we did – even though we couldn't.

Very strange.

The Officer he had just shouted at talked into a radio. The ME was enroute.

"Do you know whose it is?" I asked, incredulous that anyone could kill a newborn.

"Not yet," he replied. "But, the room up there is where she had it."

I looked up to find my partner coming out of the room, bags in hand, a look of bewilderment on his face.

"Do you have a patent down there?" he yelled.

I didn't know what to say, certainly didn't want to yell it across the lot. I started walking towards him, not wanting to look at the baby again.

"Well?" he yelled again.

"Wait," I yelled. Jim was not my regular partner, but he certainly could stand some manners training.

I approached him at the bottom of the stairway to the room of horrors.

"There's a baby in that garbage can but he's dead," I said.

"It's a *he*?" he asked.

I thought about that for a minute. I actually didn't know. You couldn't see the sex and I – well, I just assumed it was.

"Are you ok?" he asked. I appeared to be in somewhat of a stupor. "The room upstairs is a mess. Blood everywhere, especially on the bed. She must have bled like a stuck pig."

I looked at him and couldn't believe how unbelievable the entire scene was. A tiny baby was sitting – *standing* – in a garbage can and the people in this room had killed him and thrown him away like yesterday's pizza.

I went by Jim and started the slow walk up the steps. I didn't know what I would see, but I felt like, for the baby in the can, that I had to see it.

A uniformed police Officer stopped me as I approached the door.

"Your partner was already up here," he said.

"Yeah, I wanted to clear the scene and make sure he didn't leave anything."

The cop knew there wasn't anything of ours in there. He also knew there was something down there, in that garbage can, that he didn't want to see.

"Did you see him?" he asked, giving me that look. He was a father himself, I could tell.

"Yeah," I said, looking down, as if ashamed to admit it.

He studied me for a second and pulled his hand away from the door.

"Don't touch anything," he said. I walked in.

The room was, what most people would say, the typical hotel room of any number of large chain motels alongside the interstate. It was a room with colorful yellow-striped wall paper, a desk, a small chest of drawers, a round table near the front with two chairs. You could see the dressing table beyond this room, between this and the bathroom. There was a small amount of blood draining down the front of the dressing table.

There were white towels everywhere. The one exception is that they weren't all white. They were dark red, covered in old blood and – well, I didn't know what else. The smell wasn't bad, like feces – and yet, it was a dark smell. I breathed through my mouth in the hopes that smell would be reduced in my head.

The first bed had looked ruffled but not slept in.

The 2nd was where something had happened.

The blood was everywhere on the white bed sheets. The cover had been pulled back onto the floor and it was soaked in blood. A trail of blood went from that bed, along the floor, into the bathroom.

I looked towards that room and the Detective at that end of the room looked at me and shook his head.

"You don't want to go in there," he said. "More of the same. It's ugly."

I stood for a moment and tried to get what had occurred in this room.

A couple, probably teenagers (I don't know why I thought that), afraid of – what? Were they afraid of their parents, the neighbors? I honestly couldn't think of a single thing that I would be so afraid of that I would kill a baby over. She had come here, probably after going into labor. The pain, I imagined, was unlike anything she had had in her young life and both, teens or not, were terribly afraid.

How they got from there, from two people in love to two scared people, huddled in a strange hotel room, alone except for each other – and their baby. At some point in that time, they would decide to kill the baby they were bringing into the world.

How would that work, I wondered? Most babies weren't stillborn, no matter what the movies said. Most were born alive. Within seconds of the delivery, the baby would start crying – and then what? Put a wet towel over the baby's mouth until they stopped breathing? Strangle the baby to cut off the noise? What possible evil could be pushed out of someone's soul to kill a baby?

The Detective put his hand on my shoulder. "You ok?" he asked.

"Yeah," I sighed. "Do we know who did this?"

"It's a dead baby down there, isn't it?" he asked. I realized he hadn't been down to the gray garbage can without a lid.

"Yeah," I said. "Horrible."

"White male and female," he read from his pad. "About 16-17, came in for one night, left early morning, no noise, no trouble, paid in cash." We both stopped for a moment and looked at each other.

"I hope they catch the bastards," he said.

I started to walk back to the unit, down the stairs, as I saw the ME's vehicle arrive. The Officer near the can directed him over to it and pointed down, much like he had done with me. The ME looked down, asked something of the Detective and then reached down, picked him up out of the can and placed him on a black plastic body bag he had laid down.

It was a boy. He looked about 8 pounds and some ounces, blonde hair – and lifeless.

The Medical Examiner stood up and looked down at the lifeless baby for a moment. Everyone stopped what they were doing, no matter what it was, and looked in that direction.

And, at the next moment, the baby was covered by the bag.

Gone from sight. Everything went back to movement. The ME got a kit out to do some tests, the cops started to gather evidence, people started to walk away. I went back to the unit and got in, feeling as if the entire day was going to be dark.

"Pretty ugly, eh?" my partner said.

"Yeah," I said.

They say in this business that it's best not to get attached to the patients. The machine you build inside of you allows you to care, at that moment, and when that moment is over, to dump that memory, those feelings, until the next one. It is somewhat hard at times, considering the level of emotion in some calls.

This one was definitely going to be one of those.

Every day, when I pass by one of those gray, non-descript, flip door, top-rounded garbage cans, I think of that baby. I remember the day, sunshine and beautiful, a wonderful day to be born. I think about the parents of that baby, whether they are caught, arrested, tried, or whether society felt "sorry" for them and felt it was our fault, or some such silliness.

It was just a garbage can.

The Top ~~10~~ 9 truths about EMS leadership

As I rounded the hall, I could see my office and who was inside.

The next sentence will tell him, if he chooses to read this, who I am talking about. I try to keep real names out of this, but some lessons need to be taught with some specify.

As I entered my office, he was sitting in *my* chair at *my* desk.

Now, don't get me wrong. I'm not one of those "I am King" kind of guys. I just hadn't seen anyone other than myself sitting there, and it took me aback. He was spinning around, the way a child might in one of those old time soda fountains.

What he said next really threw me for a loop.

"So," he asked as he spun around in my chair. "What do you think?"

"I could do your job, you know," he continued.

I calmly (who are we kidding) told him to get out of my chair.

No, that's not what happened.

"Get up," I growled loudly. He wasn't sure if I was serious.

"I said GET UP," I shouted. He stood up immediately.

He stood up quickly, surprised by my abrupt tone.

"You have no idea what it takes to fill that chair," I stated. "You like the *style* of the shirt but you don't want to do the work it takes to wear it."

"Sorry," he sheepishly said. "I didn't know you were so touchy about that."

Actually, I didn't either.

He was a good Paramedic, one with great patient care skills, both human and technical. He was very skilled at finding out the puzzles that were our patients and focusing on the care and skills needed to make patient comfortable. His people skills with the sick patients were amazing.

What he did not have, however, was leadership skills. He "thought" he did, but friends like myself, had told him that he had to work on some people skills with non-patient folks before he could even think of being a leader in the industry.

We remain friends to this day and I don't think he took my ticked off manner as anything other than a bad day, however, I continue to keep that in my mind as a pinnacle point for future leaders.

I'm not sure if he ever got that.

In my role as both a leader and a teacher (and often I don't think you can separate the two), I have found my share of people who think they want to lead – who believe they want to "be like me."

When I give my lecture on the top 10 things a leader needs to be successful, I often think of that time. I was originally going to call this chapter "**The top 10 things you need to be a successful EMS leader**" and then I changed it to 9 because one of my closest friends, a fellow EMS leader and my mentor, Ray Graham, had disproved one

So, it came to be, at least in my mind, that being a great leader had nothing to do with WHAT you were leading but HOW you were leading. All of the things we would think you need to be a great clinician, people skills, ability to communicate, to keep your head when everyone around you is losing theirs, are skills needed for leadership.

For those of us who have been around Doctors, Nurses and/or Paramedics, we must admit that some don't have a few (and some don't have any) of those skills needed.

So, let's talk about what I think you need to be a successful leader.

~~# 10   You must be a certified Paramedic or EMT in order to properly lead EMS personnel.~~

This was the one that Ray disproved. As a former CIA operative (really, he was a Hospital Administrator but worked for the CIA), he knew no more about EMS than "sticky-side-down" for the Band-Aid, and he kept it that way. However, he did hire the right kind of people and then, left them to get the job done. I have tried to follow his lead since then. The team he created where I now was the Director turned out to be one of the first County-wide, and foremost professional EMS systems in the country.

So much for # 10.

9 – Be Yourself

So many people are promoted up the chain until they think they ARE what they DO. The rank (Lieutenant, Captain, Major, Colonel, General or whatever) gets in the way of leading. While it is true that people will treat you differently after you are promoted to a higher rank, the initial act of respect is usually ONLY out of respect for the position. The long-term respect is *earned* for a different reason. If you were honest, friendly, communicative, a people person, logical and just (notice, I didn't use the term fair – that's what you pay the bus driver), you simply have to keep those tools as you rise through the ranks. Don't be someone you think they want you to be; be who you are. You'll gain better respect and cooperation from a majority of your folks and that will be long lasting.

One caveat; they may have to change what they call you from a first name to a title (Don became Mr. Lundy in many circles). That doesn't mean they can't call you by your first name when you are discussing something privately, however, in a group, respect is calling them by their official name or title; Showing off is calling the leader by his first name. It is disrespectful to them, to the organization and to your co-workers.

#8 – Be Vulnerable

So many leaders think they have to be *perfect* in their decision and actions. The four biggest words you can use to gain respect are, "I made a mistake." When you messed something up, admit it and move on. When something upsets you, let them know it. That doesn't mean you have to blow up or yell. It simply means you are human. Because you are.

7 – Have a passion about your mission

It's hard to believe that some people actually hate their work and go there every day with a dread that could be cut with a knife. They complain about everything they are asked to do, about their pay, their working conditions, even what they have to wear (no matter whether the employer pays for it or not). I couldn't imagine going through life hating what I did – so I never have.

In EMS, it's a little different. No one does it for the money; They don't do it for the great working hours (24 hours on, sometimes, 36) or the fantastic benefits (many EMS providers still struggle to have any kind of medical insurance, retirement, etc.).

No, they do this because of a passion; one to do the right thing for someone who is in need. Realizing that if they don't do something to help someone, there is a good chance that no one will, They go through a great deal of education and sacrificing family time to learn everything they can about illness and injury so, if called, they can save someone's life.

If you are one in EMS who groans when an emergency call becomes mundane, or simply don't like it anymore unless it is a triple car versus train crash, then you've lost your passion – and you MUST get it back in order to do this job right.

Now, once you become a leader – is your passion still about the patient? Absolutely. Although it doesn't seem like it, everything you're going to deal with has to do with patient car; gas bills, tires, batteries, accessories, medication, Human Resources (the new name for Personnel) issues, disciplinary challenges, schedules – it should all focus on excellence in patient care.

Passion is not something you "get." You have it inside of you and throughout your career, in whatever it is that you are going to do, you must focus it and use it every day, to make a difference for you and the ones you lead. They can see your passion everyday if you show it to them.

They say that if you find something you love to do, you'll never work a day in your life. I love what I do, always have, and have never felt like it was work.

#6 – As a leader, your time-line changes. Unlike your role in patient care, you usually are no longer in a hurry. Slow down, work the problem. You must be thinking ahead and outside the box

A leader is constantly challenged by areas and issues that couldn't have been thought of previously. When that happens in the medical field, it is usually a quick decision that needs to be made to save the patient's life.

However, in leadership, most decisions can be handled in a timely fashion – sometimes days and sometimes longer. There's no hurry. As a leader, you must take the global approach to a problem. After all, you aren't making a decision on how to fix something in your unit – you're making it for the entire agency.

Think slow, think thorough, and think outside the box. Ask your folks what they think "we" should do and then listen to them when they give you an answer. You'll be amazed at the talent that is standing around you.

#5 – Stand up for your co-workers

This is probably one of the scariest parts of being a leader. All of us expect to make mistakes – but we want our leaders to stand with us, not making the mistake ok but, at least, not letting others beat us over the head. The leader will have their chance to do that; If there is an issue (and especially if it is public), you should let them know that you are standing with them.

Don't be concerned when some don't hear that, and decide you are not helping them. We had a serious issue in our agency involving holiday time. Working with the County, our holiday pay changed from an hour-for-hour payment (12 hour shift got 12 hour holiday) to an 8 hour holiday for those who worked it. However, we <u>did</u> keep holiday pay – and considering that the neighbor County next door had NO paid holiday pay for their EMS system (the only part of the County government who did not pay that benefit too), we felt this was a good thing. Some folks thought I had "sold them out" and that I could have kept the old holiday pay schedule "if I had wanted to." As a leader, you know the truth and, if you don't have thick skin to take the hits, you should think about doing something else with your life.

I knew the truth and I have always stood up for my employees, even when it was unpopular, even when I got suspended for it (yes, I did – but that's a story for another book).

Is this easy? Absolutely not. Politically comfortable? No. But, it's the right thing. The minute you, as a leader, let employees take a hit because you want to "save your job."

Well, as I have said to many people, "selling shoes ain't bad".

#4 – Be Forgiving

When someone makes a bone-head mistake, do you fire them for it? I have always said no, because we are human and humans are going to make mistakes.

Having said that, I know there are five areas which are not "mistakes." They are purposeful things that are done to either promote an agenda or hide the breaking of a law; lying, stealing, cheating, using illegal drugs and abusing patients. Those are my five "draw the line" areas in which people in my world can get fired on a first-time event. Those aren't "bonehead" decisions and are not tolerated.

Everything else, generally, can be dealt with by trying to change someone's behavior. Sometimes it works, sometimes it doesn't.

However, being forgiving is being human. Yes, it is somewhat painful; especially when someone makes the same mistake over and over (you may go to a termination if they can't learn from their mistakes).

As a leader, your goal is to teach those who want to lead that they are *not* infallible.

3 – Have Integrity

Integrity is a funny thing. Most that have it and have had it forever. That's because their parents, or a mentor, taught them that *everything* you do in your life rides with you forever.

Many young people believe there is a time when nothing you do really matters. That time, for many, is when you are in school. While I would agree that there are many things that could be accomplished without much of a dent in your integrity, there are a few that stay with you throughout your life.

- **Arrests** – Yes, I know that in this country, you are innocent until proven guilty in a court of law, judged by a group of your peers. If you were to move into an apartment complex and the landlady were to tell you that a rapist lived next door, what would you think? Probably, you would ask whether they were properly found guilty in a court of law by a jury of their peers (NOT). Integrity is everything.

  In the case of an employer, he does <u>not</u> need to have a jury of their peers to convict anyone of anything. In the real world of work, they have thousands who are looking for work. If you have a smear on your record, they *could* take a chance on you – but the probabilities are weak. It is not because you were or were not found guilty. It's because your integrity is in question.

- **Poor work record**- Yes, I know your former boss may have been a jack wagon – or you could have taken advantage of the company in which you may not have liked their employment opportunities. Did you come to work on time, *every day*? Were you a problem-free employee, able to take on extra work, or at least smile and say only good things about them? If not, your *integrity* may be what they don't want to buy.
- **It's not stealing – honest** – Yes, you do earn your sick and annual leave hours. You work hard for them – but, taking a sick day EVERY Friday you work is simply abuse to your co-workers and your patients. Integrity – Even when you're not there, it's there.

#2 – Have Balance

We all know people who were Mr. or Ms. EMT – someone who lived and breathed EMS. While we might think that is the way, someone eventually suffers. Not having friends outside of your work circle makes for a dull life and eventually gets in the way of your family. You must have other interests – not drinking – but baseball, church work, volunteering, wood work, fishing – anything that breaks you away from work and gets you focused on your life – which you should do.

You've heard from co-workers children who have told you, "Dad didn't make my game last week – he was working."

The children aren't telling you that to feel sorry for them. They're hoping you'll go hit the parents on the head (figuratively speaking) and tell them what they are missing.

#1 – NEVER take yourself too seriously

Many a leader I have met felt that they were wearing their "career" on their collar. His or her rank was *who they were* and, at some point, they could no longer take themselves as just another Joe who was doing a job.

Remember – at a brush of a pen, we can all lose our jobs. You don't have to do anything wrong (believe me, I have some factual data on this). It can just happen.

And, those who take themselves too seriously don't do very well.

Well, those are the 9 truths to being a successful leader in EMS. There's no magic bullets there, nothing you can *sink your teeth into*. It's being a leader enough to know that you sometimes can do great things – and being human enough to know you are human.

Dear Mom;

I know this letter may come some 40 years late, but I was just thinking of the last time we had talked.

You remember – in the Hospital after your second hip replacement. Boy, you were doing so well. It seemed that your first replacement had taken so well. You were walking well and, with the exception of the pain from the most recent one, your health had improved quite a bit. This second replacement was going to be a piece of cake.

You and I had talked just a few days after the surgery and you had mentioned that the Doctor was very pleased that both of your legs were almost even, something that evidently didn't happen too much in that type of surgery at the time. You told me that Dad was going to pick you up Sunday and bring you home.

Sunday. That day turned out not quite what we had asked for.

During that conversation, I told you about my new job as an Ambulance dispatcher. You seemed relieved. Yes, I knew you weren't too happy about the possibility that I might one day be a police Officer. Barb had told me about how you worried, so I was pleased to be able to relieve you of that worry.

You asked if I needed any money. Mom, you always asked that, as if I was a pauper. I have a job you know – a good paying one, working for a large hotel chain as a private investigator. I get two pay checks (one from the job we worked and one from the hotel chain who hired me). The hours aren't that great, but I was just beginning.

It's nice you would ask, though. I know you probably have a $20 hidden somewhere in the Hospital room.

I had interviewed for the job of dispatcher with a private Ambulance service. I met that guy named "doc" and I was really surprised when you mentioned that you knew him – in fact, you both had dated before you met Dad. I must say it took me some time to process that idea that my Mom dated! I know that sounds silly but I just never thought of it.

They hired me and started me out ten cents more than the starting pay. That meant I was making $1.60 an hour! Man, how did I fall into such a GREAT paying job?! One month later, the County bought the company and they announced that our hourly rate would go to $3.30 an hour. At that point, I'm sure we had hit the jackpot!!! That didn't even count the benefits (To tell you the truth, I didn't even know what benefits meant but I liked the sound).

And, then, there was Sunday. The day you were to go home.

I got the telephone call from Dad.

I had just gotten home from a night shift with the steel company I was working in for the investigative organization. When I came into the apartment, I heard the telephone ringing. I turned the corner to the bedroom and saw Barb sitting on the bed, with a terrible look on her face. She said the phone had been ringing like that since about 4 AM. She didn't want to answer it because – well, now, I'm sure you know why.

Yes, Mom, it's true. Barb and I were living together. I'm not sure if you ever figured that out. We went to great pains for you and Dad not to know. I loved Barbara so much, Mom. I knew she was the one. As I write this, we will have been married since 1974.

Anyhow, when Dad told me you had died, you know what happened to the men in the Lundy family. Life stopped, all images in our heads turned from color to black and white, our hearts turned to stone and there wasn't anything we didn't hear, smell or look at that didn't remind us of you. The void you left was large and unfillable. Dad – well, you know now because you are most likely together (although I am not sure if he had enough "credits" to make it to the upstairs room). Dad was pretty much useless as any husband who lost a spouse would be - but surprisingly sober.

Your funeral continues to be one of the most beautiful they had ever had in that area. There were so man flowers. The Funeral Home had never seen so many for one person. It was beautiful to see the lives you had touched but, for us, it was a very sad time.

Now, I look back at all that has happened think how proud you would be. Your son is the Director of the greatest EMS service in the nation (and of course, very humble of his folks). Mom, you would like everyone here. They take their job very seriously (like you would), love life (like you have) and laugh whenever they can (like you did). They are respective of their patients and always give the best of care. It's like working in a heavenly place.

Your daughter-in-law is a kindergarten teacher by trade. She has either been involved as a helper or the teacher in forming hundreds of small minds. She is wonderful with children, especially our son, your grandson, Robert. Throughout my career, I tried to either have a shift that would accommodate his play schedule at school and his baseball schedule later in his teen years (or switch shifts with someone). But Mom, Barbara was so good with him and continues to be. She is a Mom's Mom.

Anyhow, I never did get into law enforcement, except for a short stint in the Army. I wouldn't have liked it as a career, but it certainly gave me a view of the brave men and women on our streets that make our cities safe every day.

I just wanted you to know that Walker and I miss you every day. Every time I see someone making something from scratch (the way you used to make those lemon trees and Christmas ornaments), I think of you. I hope Heaven is busy because I know you didn't like to sit around.

One day, hopefully, we'll get to see each other again. What a great day that will be!

I'll see you later then.

Your son,

Don

Fired

I supposed every man goes through life and wonders if he is going to be fired.

I don't mean he thinks he has done something wrong – although he may have – but most men wonder, at one time or another, what would happen if they lost their job.

I used to think people didn't *get fired* but they did get *themselves* fired (I don't know where I heard that, but it sounded good).

I learned one day that it isn't always the case.

It was a very typical Friday, one with sunshine, blue skies and the usual number of calls. I was an EMS Director in the system and we were on the way to doing some great things.

Not that they hadn't already done great things. This was a system that wasn't associated with any Fire Department, one known as a "third service", who had improved their patient care and response times in the County. We had opened a new station, expanded care and improved conditions. The budget was in check, vehicles were all working – life was good.

Around 11 AM, a call came from the County Administrators office. His secretary told me Dick, Mr. Dick Waddell, wanted to see me at 1 PM. As anyone would say, I said I'd be there.

As I hung up, I had no inkling that anything was wrong. We had been nominated for a National Association of Counties award for our great work and, I assumed he wanted an update on the process. I called my wife, asked if she wanted to have an early lunch, grabbed the award application and notes, and headed out for some lunchtime lasagna.

We used to eat at a small Italian restaurant, one in a strip mall, which had tremendous lasagna. Our younger son, Robert, was 10 years old and doing well in school. My wife was off on this Friday from her position as kindergarten director at a local private school.

As I headed off to see the boss, I kissed Barbara and told her I would see her that night.

Heading up the highway, I listened to EMS radio system. It seemed quiet, not dead, but not busy. This was a Friday at the height of the winter season, so that was somewhat a blessing. After 5 PM, I knew it would pick up.

Arriving on the fourth floor of the administration building, I noted that most of the offices in that wing were empty. *It looks like lots of Friday flu*, I thought to myself. Dick came out of his office and greeted me.

"Hi Don," he said. "Come on in."

I noted he was wearing his suit jacket. That was unusual, but maybe he had just come back from a meeting.

As I settled into my chair in front of his desk, I noted he didn't take his suit jacket off as he sat behind his desk.

"Don," he said. "There is no easy way to say this."

And, with that beginning, he began to tell me that there were various people who weren't happy with my work.

"Who?" I asked.

He told me that was no concern to me and that the mere issue of people being unhappy with my performance was the issue.

"But, Mr. Waddell," I said. "My performance appraisals are all 4's and 5's, the highest ranking I can get."

"This has nothing to do with performance appraisals," he stated. I think he was about to say that it had to do with performance but realized how stupid that would sound.

"This issue with the Medical Directors has gotten them upset," he stated.

About four months earlier, the County administrator had bent to the will of the private Hospital in the area when they whined that they felt having a Medical Director who was an employee of one of the three area Hospitals (not theirs) gave that Hospital an unfair advantage.

Their answer was pretty crazy; rotate the Medical Directors between the three Hospitals every two years.

You can imagine what I thought of that idea.

"We have protocols," I explained. "They are signed by the Medical Director. The State doesn't recognize when you have three Medical Directors unless all of them sign onto the protocols."

"We have an answer to that," the one Doctor said. "We'll *vote* on the protocols every two years."

Ahhh, yes. Patient care by proxy. Lovely.

"Well, Mr. Waddell," I stated. "I still don't think that is a good idea for the system, but whatever you say; you know I'm a team player."

"Well, there's another issue," he continued. "County Council has decided to merge the EMS and Fire Departments together."

The other shoe dropped. The Fire Department had attempted a few years back to take control of the EMS system.

That had been mentioned a few years back, during a budget hearing, the two systems merging and forming one. The word "take-over" was used during the impromptu presentation.

"Chief," I asked the Fire Chief in front of the Budget Committee. "How many calls do you run in the fire service?"

"About 1200 a year," he said, proud of that accomplishment.

"Well," I said, scratching my chin in front of the public finance meeting. "We ran 10,000 last year, so, yeah, I think it's possible we could absorb the Fire Department without hurting our operation."

It was not the answer he was looking for. Of course, the elected folks really didn't care *who* absorbed *who* so it was nothing to them what occurred.

However, to the Fire Chief, who saw this takeover as increasing calls (we would call it *call-counting*) thereby increasing jobs in the Fire Department, it did not appear to be a position he was warming up to.

"I think we should get together and discuss this further before bringing it back to you guys," he said to the Committee in his heavy NY accent.

With that, it ended. It was never brought up in a meeting or hearing again.

But, I knew it wasn't the end.

The truth of the matter was that the great work fire service had done in developing fire-proof materials and building codes, putting sprinkler systems in commercial buildings, handing out smoke alarms and other fire reducing items, reduced the need for such a labor-intense organization, or so it seemed to some politicians.

You certainly couldn't justify 4-5 men on a fire truck when fires were down 80%. Jobs were at stake.

On the other end of the spectrum was EMS, Busy, busy, like a one-armed paper hanger and it didn't seem to be wearing off. *Everyone* needled EMS.

With some Fire Departments doing great as the primary EMS provider, it's obvious that all Fire Departments didn't start by a takeover like what was being proposed in our town. Many had no separate EMS agency and poor EMS service and they decided to expand their role so that patient care could be established. However, in our case, EMS had been established some years ago as a third service and was running great.

For our Fire Department, it involved finding our Fire Department a mission. At this moment, the mission appeared to be EMS focused.

Dick was looking at me after mentioning that and I realized I hadn't commented.

"Well," I said, realizing that this was a done deal. "As I said, I think you know how I feel about that, but you're the boss, so whatever you say goes. What do you want me to do to help in this changeover?" I had pulled my pen and pad of paper out to take notes.

"Well," he said. "The first thing I need is the keys to your car. You're fired."

I looked up in utter shock. I don't think anyone had said anything that was more surprising to me than that. I also did something I had never done before, or since.

I cursed in the boss's office.

"What the F**K are you talking about?" I yelled.

"We only need one Chief and I already have one," he said, smiling.

"But you're Chief doesn't know a thing about running EMS," I said. I immediately worried about the system and what effect it would have on the employees.

"No problem," he said. "He'll pick it up."

My shock wore off and I started to realize about logistics.

"Are you going to drive me to the office to get my things?" I said in as calm of a voice as I could muster. "I didn't come here thinking I was going to be fired for doing my job!"

Dick hadn't thought of that. You could tell that he was thinking. He didn't want to have me sit in his car for the 10 minute ride down to the EMS office. "No, you should drive the car back to headquarters and gather your things."

He went on to say that he had decided to pay me six months' severance pay, but I didn't hear him. I stood up, exited his office and realized that NO ONE was on the floor. Obviously, this wasn't the case of the Friday flu. He had told folks they didn't want to be there for what was to follow.

As I drove back, I was truly numb. I didn't hear the radio, didn't think about traffic, and didn't know where I was going. I arrived back at the office and went directly to my office, closing the door.

The first call I made was to my wife. I told her what had happened and that I needed her to come down to pick me up.

The 2nd call I made was to my brother. By that time, I was crying.

I know we must have talked for about 30 minutes and I truly don't remember most of the conversation (sorry Walker). I do remember, however, the one thing he told me.

"Remember, Don," he said. *"It's their mistake, not yours."*

My wife arrived at the same time that the Fire Chief did. His face looked worried, sad, somehow surprised. He tried to say something to me. I asked him to stay out for a minute.

Barb came in with Robert and both hugged me. The three of us walked out together.

As we were pulling away, Robert asked why they didn't want me working there anymore. I told him I didn't know. That is when it happened.

Robert said he had some money saved up in his bank and that I could have it if I needed it. I started to cry again and did so all the way home.

The following day, Saturday, we spent at the Little League tryouts. The newspaper headlines had let everyone know my condition that weekend (EMS Director fired, no reason given) and, twice, Robert came to the fence, saw my sad face and told me that the next hits were for me.

I do remember that he hit them hard and far!

The following days were very unusual. We found that some of who we thought were close friends, stayed away as if we had the plague. We also got phone calls from people who we thought weren't that close, offering help if we needed it.

The worst part, to me at least, was Sunday. The supposed "Christians" in the church, who wouldn't talk to us, wouldn't even acknowledge that our life was about to fall apart simply blew me away. It gave me a taste of the church that I haven't gotten over to this day.

That Monday, we bought a 2nd car, on credit, and upon our return home, we started to see a small sliver of hope. On the answering machine were seven job offers. While that was satisfying, I had wanted to return to school to get my degree and thought this was the perfect time. So, after three months of being paid for not going to work (another strange feeling), I accepted a position with Greenville County EMS in South Carolina. They had a school program that paid for you to attend school and had a very impressive system! That program allowed me to get my Associates degree in EMS and my Bachelor's degree and, eventually, through all of that, to work with three of the most authentic, professional EMS systems in the nation.

So, for those who have not been fired in a job (especially "without cause"), a few thoughts; was it rough for those first months? Oh, yes. Scary? Absolutely. What kept us going was that we loved each other and we knew God had a plan. While it is true that Barbara wasn't very happy about the plan, including her move from Florida where her parents spent half of their year and where all of our friends were, but she morphed and enjoyed it eventually. We made new friends and found some old friends who lived near there. We also found a tremendous church home (Thanks Mike) that fed us every week, so that we kept the dream alive. We knew, eventually, we would see what this was all about.

We did. After getting my degrees, I was hired as Director for one of the most professional EMS systems in the nation. The people I work with every day are awesome. We received the State's top system of the year award and was named National EMS System of the Year for 2010.

For the 2nd time, I received The EMS Director of the Year award.

Walker, you were right. It WAS their mistake!

So, you may be wondering what happened to the other service? I am pleased that they have merged and run successfully today, as one Fire/EMS system. I wasn't very pleased to see billboards posted at each end of the County telling visitors that their lives are in danger because the County Administration won't work with the union and, because of that, it is dangerous to live, work and/or drive there. Later, I learned that, due to a billing error by the Fire Department, they had to pay a fine in excess of $300,000 to the Federal Government.

I guess the idea of *"he'll pick it up"* was an expensive lesson.

Today, I tell folks that I think everyone should be fired once in their life. I also tell them that friends who they think are close may not be and friends who are distant may be very close. Above all, the power of love and the family will get you by and make you strong.

The next adventure will be tremendous!

STEMI

It started like – well, many of my patients would say – indigestion.

When I go back and really think about it, it was anything but indigestion – but my "denial" gene had initially decided that is probably what it was.

My wife and I had just finished a great meal at one of our local, popular barbeque restaurant (as they say, you can't swing a dead cat in South Carolina without hitting a barbeque joint) and, as I went out into the cold air, I suddenly felt as if I was going to faint. It passed quickly and I blamed it on the temperature change that night.

As I reached the rear of the car, about 20 steps from the door of the restaurant, it started. It was pain – *and burning*. Burning like I had never had before, so hot that I thought if I touched my chest, I would burn my hand.

I rubbed my chest (you would think by then I would realize it wasn't what I thought it was) and told Barb I was uncomfortable. I opened the door, sat in the driver's seat, and the pain hit me like a ton of bricks.

No – it really wasn't pain. It was a fire – but it *hurt*. I didn't understand what was happening; only that it wasn't going away. In fact, it was getting much, much worse. By the time I settled into the seat, I felt like my chest was going to burst into flames.

I thought, i*t was the worst feeling I had ever had.*

It **was** the worst feeling I had ever had.

Barb asked if I wanted her to drive (I, of course, thought she meant to home – she had other ideas) and just as I said no, just when I thought it couldn't get any worse, the fire/pain increased to an unbearable heat.

What in the world is going on? I wondered. *What would hurt this much?*

I suddenly felt air hunger. I had only read of it before now, and, of course, seen patients who had it. I had treated many patients who were "short of breath" with their gasping, but you couldn't really *see* air hunger. It was that I wasn't having hard time breathing – I just felt I needed air.

I opened the driver's door and swung my legs out to the outside. The fire was unbearable and I felt like I had a 500 pound weight on my chest. The weight on my chest was a dead giveaway (no pun intended), but I still hoped it wasn't that.

And then, I had the strangest feeling. I can't explain to you what it is or how it came into my head, but it was as strong as any thought I had in quite some time.

I looked straight up at my wife, who had come around to the driver's side.

"I think I'm going to die," I cried.

I think I'm going to die. The *feeling of impending doom* I had read about and taught all of my former students.

"Make the call!" I told her. She knew what that meant.

…………………..

If any of you stand in your kitchen and look at your refrigerator, in many instances, you would look at a poster board history of your family, especially if you have children or grandchildren. The refrigerator is the advertisement for some of the finest art, travel brochures and general life involving small children, dogs, long-lost relatives and who is important in their lives, as well as situations, celebrations, life-changing events in your life.

Our refrigerator is like that.

It is one week since my heart attack. I am standing in our kitchen and the quietness of the morning is only broken by Lilly, our golden retriever/greyhound who wants to go out – again! I ignore her for a minute and stare at the refrigerator. I immediately see the picture of our son, taken at graduation at FSU. How did *that much time fly by?* Then, my eyes move to the group standing in front of the boat we took on our 25th wedding anniversary. I also realized that two of the eight in the picture were no longer with us. How did *that* happen?

Memories, magnetized on a metal box. Who would imagine that so much of your life could be shown on such a small piece of metal?

I wasn't sure, but I think the medical issue that happened in the past week almost made me one of those magnets.

I can't even write it out unless I think hard so as not to cry. It was an MI – Myocardial Infarction, what laypeople would know as a heart attack. That really was what it was. It just doesn't seem like that should happen to someone as – well, as healthy as I am. I don't drink, don't smoke, don't' inject anything (I don't like needles – I am allergic to pain) and eat as right as anyone can without going over the cliff. What was I doing in a bathrobe looking at this metal marvel, in review of things I had lived through and thinking…..well, what if that had all ended? A scary thought.

…………………………

Barbara tells the 911 operator that she needs an Ambulance. She tells them the restaurant we are at but she doesn't know the exact address. Yes, she says, at the Central Mall. Then, she tells the dispatcher, "chest pain."

I hear her but I cannot look up. I continue to feel the burning – it is much worse now. I try to notice myself and what is happening. I don't feel sweaty and don't feel short of breath (as I hang out of the still car). But, mostly, I am worried about what I said to her. *I think I am going to die.* Where did THAT come from? I can't explain why I said it, but I did mean it. The feeling was still there. I have to say -

I wasn't panicked – I wasn't even scared. It was sort of a statement of fact. But, why would I say that.

I think of my son, when I talked to him last – *what did I say to him?* There is so much I want to say and do and not enough time.

Time. That's what was running out.

It seems like only 40 seconds or so that Barb is on the phone when I hear a siren in the distance. *That's them, I think.* They are close and that is a good thing. I might pass out at any minute and I need to stay awake to tell them what is going on.

I need to stay awake? Why would I think that? What is going on?

. . . .

Just below the center of the center of the refrigerator, I see the drawings of our foster child in South America, the bigger picture of him grown at 18. We were members of an organization that helps children in South America and, from what we could tell, much had helped this once small child into teen and eventually manhood.

I wondered what happened to those in that country who suddenly had chest pain. Did they have a system like ours? Unlikely, but, still, I wondered.....

. . . .

As I look up in my tears, my heat ripping through my chest, I see Alex. He's been a Paramedic with me for about 2 years or so. Behind him is his partner, Mallory. Alex has a calm face and demeanor about him. Although Mallory is smiling, she is moving – as I would say – with purpose, rather quickly and getting the equipment set up.

I tell Alex my chief complaint and, after a few simple questions, he moves me over to the stretcher. As I do so, Barbara asks if I want to give her my wallet and phone. I do so and the crew gets me settled onto the litter. As I lay back, I realize I can't lay flat and ask to sit up. They sit the back of the bed up and I get to watch the symphony unfold.

Alex and Mallory are moving the stretcher around to the rear of the unit. I can see the car, door still open. A fire truck is pulling up. Mallory smiles at me as if we are about to start a discussion on a book. Calm and confident.

Behind Mallory, my wife continues to have a calm voice. She still is smiling but focused towards what is happening to me. The Ambulance door closes and I hear Mallory tell Barb she will get her seated in the front. Alex is getting me on oxygen and Mallory is getting the wires to the EKG ready. I feel the oxygen blow into my nostrils and I start to breathe it. Immediately, the fire subsides a little.

I think it is at that point that I knew I was in trouble (Yeah, I know, *what took you so long?*). I think to myself, oxygen doesn't reduce indigestion. It does reduce cardiac pain.

Ok, well, the fire is reduced and I'm still awake. All good things.

"Don't worry Mr. Lundy. You're in good hands" Alex tells me. His face is still calm. That means the world to me right now. As long as they aren't panicked, I'm not panicked.

I focus on the picture of our 35th wedding anniversary party. We had invited eight of our closest friends to a dinner cruise with us, complete with limo, leaving from the hotel where we were celebrating and returning later that night. My brother, Walker and his wife Saralyn, Cliff and Jackie, Tracy and Scott and Ray and Jane, all close friends and family! What a wonderful group of people!

Walker and I are 10 years and 4 days apart, birthday wise. He has always been a superb older brother, raising me for most of my life. The most talented Editor in newspaper's history (ok, so I'm a little biased), he has not hesitated to be there when needed – to be an ear that I could bitch and yell at – and someone who, on most days, makes much more sense than the average bear. His wife is originally from Atlanta Georgia, a wonderful partner in life for him and a fantastic friend to us and to everyone she meets. I have to brag and say she is one of those women who could take a cup of flower and three safety pins and create a beautiful 5 course meal for 20, without so much as blinking her eye! She is much like my mother that way.

Cliff was my Safety Officer shortly after arriving at Charleston County EMS. The current safety Officer there was in ill health and, following his retirement, Cliff applied for the job and clearly beat any other candidates. He was *made* for this job. I had known Cliff about five years before, when I had become Director in Orangeburg County. He was one of the friendliest people in that circle. He was the Assistant Director for Colleton County EMS. After the announcement of my moving to Charleston, his wife, Jackie, a realtor, helped us purchase our home there. We have been life-long friends since.

Tracy is now the Director for medical affairs at the Greenville County Detention Center. Once a Paramedic Supervisor, she was my boss when I arrived in Greenville, a demoted EMS Director who wasn't sure I could ever do the job on the street after five years of driving a desk. Tracy treated me with respect, demanded excellence from me and showed me that I could do whatever I wanted to do if I wanted to do it. She is one of the sharpest Paramedics I have ever met. She met and married her life partner, Scott, and we were honored to be one of the invited few to see that happen. I think she is the only bride that I ever cried for when I saw her coming down the aisle. Believe me, they were tears of joy.

Ray Graham was the EMS Director for Charleston County EMS when I first arrived in Orangeburg. A former CIA operative, he is the most interesting characters I had ever met, a close friend, a father figure for me and a tremendous EMS leader. He had been retired about two years when the picture was taken but he looked just as young as he did when I first met him. Jane and he met while he was working at Charleston County and she has been his constant companion ever since. She is a good Shepherd for him (since he can decide to do some pretty wild things at times, like run in Pamplona "running of the bulls" – yes the REAL one and he eventually did!).

As I look at that picture on our metal life frame, I realize the reality that, as that picture is taken, two of the people in it will not be with us within four years of that night. Cliff will be diagnosed with Pancreatic Cancer and be dead within 4 months of finding it. Ray will develop two tumors, both cancerous. The first will be taken out successfully, the second will kill him.

Such good friends. Such good times.

………………..

I listen to Alex when he looks at me and then looks at the Electrocardiograph (EKG). I ask him to tell me the truth and he does.

"There are some ST changes in your EKG, sir", he says, still with a smile and calmness that helps me immensely. "We're going to call a STEMI."

I knew what S-T changes were from my training. Each part of the EKG has a letter to note its location. It starts with the letter P, then QRST and finally U. Each section has a unique meaning for your heart heath. The S and T wave are right next to one another, and elevation of those two waves means trouble.

ST elevation, possible MI – or STEMI. It's terminology I had heard many times – for other patients – and a part of the system we had worked on developing in early 2002. Earlier, I had directed the first EMS system in South Carolina which transmitted EKGs to an emergency room. Charleston County was one of the first in the nation to have a concise cardiac system, complete with 12 lead EKG, an alert for the Hospital and a system that allowed most cardiac patients to go directly from the Ambulance to the cauterization lab. The process was as exciting as the process of how we got there.

After getting the three Counties and three competing Hospitals in one room, a grant was discussed which would allow the purchase of communications equipment (to send the EKG to the ER) for every Ambulance in the tri-county region?

"What are you going to do with it?" EMS asked.

"Well we'll read it," the Hospitals said. All but one.

"Well, for us, we're going to open the cath lab and direct the patient right to there, right on the Ambulance stretcher," they said.

This was heresy in the Hospital world.

All patients stopped in the ER. What if they weren't stable? After all, what was the Cauterization lab going to do for them?

After discussing it, we all agreed that hemodynamic ally (blood pressure) unstable patients would stop but most would go directly upstairs. The other Hospitals agreed.

With that decision the STEMI cardiac care program in Charleston progressed to one of the smoothest, well-run, patent-focused systems in the country. Three competing Hospitals, three "competing" counties (we were all friends, but we loved to "one-up" the others) agreed to a system that would significantly improve patient care in the region - and no one yelled at anyone!

I thought of all of that while Alex asked me if I needed any pain relief. I declined.

"Let's see if nitroglycerin helps you at all," as I lifted my tongue for a small spray of something that didn't taste bad or good. Nitroglycerin, while in some form, is used for explosives, is also used, in this formula, to open up cardiac vessels in order for more oxygen to reach this important muscle.

He told me he was going to the radio to tell them what was coming.

As Alex disappeared behind me, I looked at the interstate pass by us as the siren wailed. I hoped Barbara wasn't that upset or scared. I worried about her.

Unknown to me, she was in full responder mode. She had already called the church on her cell phone and, with siren blaring in the background, told them to put me on the prayer list.

She promptly hung up and called our local Chaplaincy group. She told them to get a Chaplain to Roper ER right away and that I was being transported for chest pain. The third call was to our *unofficial* nephew, Robert (you have these in your family – close friends since the 4th grade with his dad who is like a brother from another mother), who needed to go to the house and take care of the dog.

I didn't know any of this was happening. I heard Alex as he presented me…..

"….a 60 year old male, sub sternal chest pain, non-radiating, stable….ST elevation in V leads, estimated time of arrival is now 10 minutes."

The Hospital asked for name and a date of birth for me.

Name is Lundy, L-U-N-D-Y, first name Don………..."

There was a long pause on the radio. Alex knew what it was.

"Yes, this is the EMS Chief!"

"ooooooookay," the voice pushed out. "We'll be ready."

Alex returned to his seat next to me and we both looked at one another and chuckled. It was then I realized that behind that calm face, Alex was scared to death. The EMS Chief was on his stretcher and he was dying.

…………………..

As I took the peach tea out of the refrigerator, the door closed and I saw the "selfie" my son had taken on his first day of work at a national tax corporation. Was that really him? He was only 5 years old and a blonde, toe-headed youngster full of energy. He had a smile that would melt your heart and the energy to make you wish you had an extra set of batteries. He loved his large tricycle and, well now, he was 31 years old, taller than me, better looking than me (ok, Robert, don't get cocky) and certainly had math down to a fine science, something his Dad never did. Obviously, he had much of his Mothers talents (especially in the brains department) and when I thought of that, I smiled more.

Around the picture was an Andy the Ambulance magnet, one gotten when our first Andy the Ambulance Robot came to The Orangeburg County EMS. A State grant bought what probably was one of the best public relations tools we had there. All of the schools wanted to see Andy and figure out how he "talked" to you (compliments of a wireless headset).

To the left of the picture, there were other magnets, one from the ASPCA, where we had gotten our Husky Annie and another from the Alamo. Barb and I had visited there a few years back and were amazed when we looked to see where the tokens to the tourist were made. We had been big anti-China folks and were floored when we saw the magnet memorializing the battle that took place there – made in Mexico!

I stood, looking at that large metal magnet and paper view of my life. Where did the time go?

. . . .

I felt the unit pull into the parking area and back into the Hospital Ambulance space. The doors opened and a plethora of familiar faces looked up at me. Chuck, Donna, Bubba, the ER Nurse, all looked with a calm but serious face.

There were jokes thrown to me trying to keep me calm (that is what I would commonly do to calm others) but I don't remember any of them. I had just about talked myself into it being nothing to be worried about when the ER doc said hello to me and explained they were going to keep me on the stretcher, get a chest x-ray and take me direct to the cath lab.

….the cath lab? Aren't you even going to wait for the x-ray to see what this is REALLY about?

As the ER crew started to undress me, although they only get me from the waste up, I realized that this was probably bad (leave it up to a man to realize it's *really* serious when his clothes are ripped off). No one takes clothes off in in *that* much of a hurry unless it's bad. The Nurses are asking if I am allergic to anything, particularly pain medication. I loudly say NO and make sure everyone is aware that I am allergic ONLY to pain.

A Nurse asks me to lean forward and a cold plate of x-ray film is put behind me. Damn, that's cool!! I lay back and everyone gets out of the room who does not want to be radiated.

I make sure I'm smiling – hey, who knows who is going to see this thing?

The film is removed and I am, still on the Ambulance stretcher, pushed out of the ER room and into a hallway. Barbara is moving alongside, holding my hand. I feel I have to stay strong for her, so I smile and give her the thumbs up sign, tangled in the IV line. She doesn't smile back but gives me a look of confidence, as if she knows everything is going to be ok.

In 39 years of marriage, I have learned to trust that look. Somehow, that makes me feel much better.

. . . .

As I poured the tea, I looked back to see the picture of Tina, our first foster daughter, all grown and a mother of five, with her husband.

Barb and I had decided young in our life, to become volunteer foster parents. The program in our State dealt with all ages but we thought teenagers would be the hardest to place, so we volunteered for ages 10-17.

Tina came to us after running away from home. She was polite, well versed in manners and happy to be with us. Being new foster parents, we brought her into our lives, eating at the dining room table for dinner (we would soon learn that many kids we received had never done that), entered her in the local school system and listened as she talked about her life.

The story of her horrible home life at the hands of her stepfather would come later.

Her mother was single at the time, divorced from her father, and took every opportunity to mentally abuse her. She seemed to thrive in our home, smiling every day, enjoying school and being a normal 14 year old.

That's when the phone call came.

The case worker had requested we bring Tina and all of her belongings and that she was going home.

We were puzzled. We, nor Tina, had been to see the counselor. How could everything be ok?

We arrived at the building, all the time Tina telling us she would not go back. We asked that she be patient while we talked to the counselor.

Deloris came in and escorted Tina to another room and came back to us.

"Where are her things?" she asked, rather flatly.

From the room next door, yelling and then screaming started. One voice was Tina and, I assumed the other was her mother.

"Well," the counselor said. "She'll need those things. They've made up and her stepfather is coming back home. Everything is falling into place. She's going home today."

I looked at her in disbelief.

"Do you hear the yelling?" I asked. "Her stepfather abused her in that home!"

She looked at me with a flat face. "Well, she should have reported it when it happened," she stated. "There's nothing I can do about it now."

Both Barbara and I stood not believing what was happening.

"Isn't there anything we can do to help?" we asked.

"No," she told us. "Especially now. She'll go home and any interference you try will only make it worse."

After a few more minutes of the screaming from next door, the counselor looked at us.

"If *she* calls you," she said. "Then, you can help her – but it must be initiated from *her*."

It was as if she was talking to us in code.

Tina came out of the room, tears running down her face.

"Don't let them do this," she begged.

Now, it was time for tears from both Barb and I.

"You'll be ok," we said, not believing our own words. "Give it a try."

The room fell into silence.

"Could we have a minute with her?" we asked.

Her Mom spoke up. "Yeah, but don't try anything."

We went out into the hallway and told her what we had learned.

I looked her in the eye and with all of the sincerity of a father, said, "If it gets bad again, you can call the police." Then, I explained, "Tell them about us." We were hoping the cops would know what to do.

One week later, Tina was back in our house, happy again, and there was a counselor who had been foiled at getting rid of another case.

Later, she was adopted by a wonderful family. Years after that she married and has a fantastic family of her own.

One life of many that Barb and I hoped we changed for the better.

. . . .

I started to hear noises. . . . . . .

The elevator opens and we travel about 50 feet to the door of the cath lab and everyone is told they have to stay outside. I kiss Barb, again with that look of confidence – and peace – and the door is shut in front of them.

I am lifted onto a hard table, covered in a wonderful warm blanket (thumbs up for the guys who sell those things) and a strange man starts to unzip my pants to take them off. I lift my rear end to help them and am suddenly naked under the blanket. The Doctor is there – my new Cardiologist – and he explains what he is going to do, what will happen after and that everything is going to be ok. In the middle of that conversation, he grabs and feels for my femoral artery.

Now, at this point in the book if you do not know where that is, I invite you to Google that and you'll understand what I am about to say.

A strange man is grabbing and feeling in an area I haven't had felt by a man – EVER! I look up and realize we are going to do a cath, understand it involves a large needle – and pain – and mention to the doc that I haven't had pain medicine yet. He calmly tells me it will be on board before he starts.

He continues to grab at my groin.

The Nurse next to me gets my attention (actually getting me away from the doc so he can prepare) and asks me again what occurred?

Geez – how many people do I need to tell this to?

I explain the story to him and at the end, he asks if I was upset at the time or in an argument, or under any pressure.

No, I answer.

Then, he asks a question that is only strange in the way it sounds.

"So," he states. "There was nothing unusual that occurred?"

The reason that was so strange is that, as he asked, it sounded like he was moving away from me. I could see him, though, and he wasn't moving at all.

"Well," I said, with a sudden push of the lack of inhibition. "There was a guy trying to remove my pants, but except for that, nothing."

I watched him lean over to the doc. "Meds are on board and we're ready," he calmly said.

The lights went out.

………………….

I turned to go into the family room and glanced at one last memory on the ice box.

The cloth-line-type clip, one of many on the top left corner, held tickets to the upcoming Christmas Concert with the Men's Chorus. I had been a member of this outstanding singing group for four years and I thoroughly enjoyed each time I got to sing with them. They were 50 of the most talented guys I had ever met – and, truth be told – if we hadn't met in the chorus, I doubt many of us would know each other. We all came from different backgrounds, different lives, but we all had the love of music in us.

The group raised money for High School Chorus and/or music major scholarships.

Behind that set of tickets were other schedules of things coming up for the holidays we wanted to attend. Behind all that was an airline voucher we had planned on using on an upcoming trip. This corner of our refrigerator had become our "what's next" corner, where we put upcoming things we would or would want to do.

Here, standing in the middle of my kitchen, resting following what was to be one of the most life-changing events ever to happen to me, I was reminded how blessed I was to have Barbara, the woman in my life who continues to save me every day, and my son, Robert, who has made a Dad proud in so many way. Add my brother and his wife, my niece and nephew and their families and our friends and I realize, even with all that has happened, I am, without a doubt, the luckiest man alive.

As my brother would say, "Life is good."

……………..

I woke up in a room in ICU, two Nurses at my side on the right, my beautiful bride to my left. Everyone was smiling.

That's a good sign, eh?

"Hey Mr. Lundy," a Nurse said. "I'm Melissa and this is Karen and we'll be your Nurses for the 24 hours or so. Your cath was a complete success and the Doctor says there won't be any complications. You have to stay very still for the next 12 hours. You have a sandbag on your groin to help with the bleeding."

I was bleeding? From what?

"Here's your call button," she said. "Can we get you anything?"

Slowly, I realized that there were a gaggle of people waiting outside the door.

"Well," I said. "I feel a warm liquid in my groin dripping. Either I am having an accident or it's bleeding."

They put the blanket back only to find the dressing hasn't held well. They immediately move to redo the bandage (did I mention it REALLY stuck to everything, and I mean *everything, if you get my drift*).

Cleaned up and no longer dripping, they leave me to my wife.

"Some want to know if they can come in and see you," she says.

Why is she so garbled? She usually speaks very clearly.

"Sure," I say.

Both Chuck and Donna, my Deputy Directors of Operations and Administration, came in to see that I am fine.

Why are they garbled too? It must be me.

I ask Chuck to not put out that I had – I couldn't even say it – an *incident* is what I think I called it. Let everyone know I am ok but would rather get through ICU before we have mass visitors.

…………..

As I stood back one more time and looked at the large metal "life picture" called a refrigerator, I saw the various postcards from places we had been, magnets of famous places we had seen and experienced, pictures of friends, both here and gone, notes of things we needed to remember, tickets to future events, so many memories – and, yet, there would still be space for the future.

…………..

I remember later that night the Nurse giving me a wonderful concoction of Magnesium, which she says I was low on and is a standard drink for post heart attack patients.

There it was, that word – heart attack. Did I really have a heart attack?

I drink it (not recommended as a delicious mixture for anyone interested) and rest again.

It is 3 AM and, even though I asked for something to sleep (they gave me 5 different choices including morphine! I just wanted a *little* something – Loratab would do), I couldn't. A lot was going through my mind. Silly things, like who would succeed me in NAEMT if I didn't make it?

Who would take my job at EMS? How would I get all of my passwords to Barbara in time?

NURSE walked into the room and sets up some equipment.

"How do you feel?" she asks. I tell her I am doing fine, although I can't sleep.

"Well," she says? "Your chemistry is good and everything looks great, so we're here to take the sheath out of your leg. I brought some morphine."

I didn't know what a sheath was, why I had it in my leg, why she was going to take it out and why she only gave me one choice – Morphine.

She then explained that there was a plastic sheath inserted for the cauterization and that it remained there for 3-6 hours just in case they had to go back in. Since it was in an artery, they were going to have to put tremendous pressure on it when they pulled it out so I wouldn't bleed to death. The morphine? Well, that was to help relax me.

They gave me the morphine and, suddenly, I wondered why I was so afraid of it.

I have given morphine to hundreds of patients and many got sick to their stomach from it.

Not me.

This was the MOST WONDERFUL DRUG they had ever made. All of my achy joints (which, remember hadn't moved for several hours – but with one little drug, all of my joints felt GREAT – as did I.

They pulled the sheath and both Nurses pressed down on my groin. Now, in most situations, where two strong Nurses were pushing my entire abdominal cavity through the mattress, I would scream, in this particular case, it was all groovy.

I slept VERY well for several hours, awakening to see Barbara at my side.

She was smiling.

Within the next 36 hours, I would be moved down to a step-down unit, visited by many, including Alex, who humbly said he really didn't do much, but I corrected him and mentioned he had saved my life.

"The Doctors can't work on something they don't have," I reminded him.

Eventually, two days after having a heart attack, I was released on the day before Thanksgiving.

The Cardiologist said I should be able to lead a full life. "You were very lucky," he said. "You came to the Hospital quickly and we have an excellent EMS system here."

I knew both were true and had a tremendous reason for my good health.

As I was wheeled out of the door to my car, the fresh air I smelled took on an entirely new thought process. The sun was shining and I had been given another chance.

That Thanksgiving, we ate at one of our favorite restaurants and celebrated like never before. There was no noise, no dancing, but lots of holding hands. Lots of smiles.

In the next months, I would see my Cardiologist to get a clean bill of health. Taking Aspirin and my new blood thinner proved too much, with as much as 10 nose bleeds a day. I took Aspirin off of the list for a while, the Doctor later prescribing that I take it twice a week.

"My job," he said, "is to make sure your pipes are clear. Anything I can do to do that, I'll do."

That made sense. I had no other nosebleeds after that.

I did have a bout of depression that I couldn't explain but, evidently, everyone who has had a heart attack understands it. Sudden bursts of crying seemed to be an add-on, but I was lucky to be somewhere, somewhat private so I didn't embarrass myself.

That's a man for you; Embarrassment was worse than the chest pain.

I do have a new outlook on life. While some would say I need to "take it easy" and slow down, I disagree. I think we have led a rather exciting life, not saying no to what many would. We traveled to Washington DC a week after the 9/11 attacks. We were not going to let them win. An added bonus was that we had the entire town to ourselves and saw some of the things we would have had to stand in line for, otherwise.

We had bought a single engine airplane and learned to fly in it. We learned, with our son, to scuba dive and still enjoy that sport to this day. We travelled to quite a few countries where we barely knew the language and, in one case, got lost from each other for 12 exciting minutes.

We've ridden horses in the mountains and done white water rafting. We've camped out where a pair of eyes staring at us gave us the creeps – and all of that – ALL OF IT – I would do over again.

And, I just may.

While I do (I think) take better care of myself, I continue at the gym, rest when I can and love life like never before.

Having said that, there is no slow down. As Dr. Sally Karioth, a good friend of mine, once noted, "If Life is what you make it, then I have got to get crackin'!"

THOSE WITH A PATCH

A funny thing happened on the way to my most recent staff meeting.

Actually, it had happened weeks before. It was one of those ideas you get and sounds so good. You know *everyone* will embrace it when you tell them. You can't wait to break the exciting news.

This whole idea started flowing shortly after a department meeting that I had with the medical staff. Some of you may not know of this type of meeting, but it had been set up long ago by my predecessor and it seemed to work well.

This is how the meeting went. After an in service, all personnel from LT up were excused. All that were to attend this meeting were Crew Chiefs (Lead Paramedic) and crew members. Behind closed doors, they would have the opportunity to have a one-on-one (or some would say a fifty-on-one depending on which chair you were in – theirs or mine) with the boss. This wasn't supposed to be a "bitch" session, but a "think tank" of issues that the employees felt needed to be fixed, along with ideas on how to fix them.

I had continued the tradition with a little twist, showing up in a superman t-shirt and a sitting on my own stool. I had stopped the meetings for a while after I thought nothing was being accomplished with them. In fact, without much structure, it did turn into a bitching match without many answers to anything.

However, I was wrong about it not doing anything.

Even without the structure, many people threw out their frustrations at different areas of the department. When I had stopped, several asked that it be re-implemented. When I picked it back up, many said they enjoyed the time together. It was not a free-for-all and, in fact, helped me to gain some insight into the system from their point of view.

So, when I met with them, we had some structure and talked about the system. After that meeting, I realized that I had challenged myself.

How do I get employees morale to improve?

That question has plagued leaders for years. I have always felt that most morale came from within (or at least mine did) and that it was rare, if ever, that anyone from the outside of my life would boost my morale.

I had been talking to several leaders in the EMS field and asked them when was the last time they had been on an Ambulance was.

"As a crew member?" one asked in disbelief.

"Yeah," I said without blinking an eye.

After some eerie silence, most of them said they hadn't been on a unit in years. In fact, a few said they didn't need to be on a truck, because they had been promoted through the ranks and had "*earned*" not being on the truck. It was apparent that most had never even thought of doing something like that. After all, they had worked hard in the field at one time or another.

During the same kind of meeting the month before, we had talked about several issues, one of them being the morale of the department and what we could do to improve it. Just throwing it out there, many gave me the impression that they felt it wasn't their issue - it was "them."

They gave the impression that the problems of the department were at the root of the people who were on the street. During the conversation, one employee was talked about in reference to a problem he was having adjusting to the 24 hour shift.

One of my best (or so I thought) Supervisors lamented. "Big baby's," she said.

We had ended that management meeting with the idea pushed forward by my command staff that "they" would have to suck it up and get it done. Now, at another command staff meeting, I had to tell them the hard truth.

It wasn't *them*.

"It's us," I said calmly.

I went on to tell them that, yes, I did believe that there was much that the medical staff could do to improve their disposition regarding their workplace. However, there was also much we could do to get ours as well. One of the things, I felt, was that anyone in administration "with a patch" should ride one 12 hour shift per month, particularly during the shortage we had.

My idea was met with silence, then with anger.

One Supervisor told me that he thought the issue was that the newer people didn't understand what the current shift Supervisors had done to get to where they were. He also felt that the possibility of the Supervisor hurting themselves would be too great.

Frankly, I was flabbergasted. Here was my team of leaders making excuses as to why they wouldn't – well, LEAD. They were not going to do the same job that they were asking their personnel to do. Although they thought that since they once "did it", it should count (and I do think that should count - somewhat), I actually saw no harm in having our Managers "lead by example" instead of "exemption." Frankly, I didn't understand why they were fighting this so hard.

Then, it hit me.

When I had first decided to work a shift as a leader, it was as a third person. I realized how much I had lost in skill level and knowledge and frankly, I was scared to death. I don't think I showed it (good acting skills) but I desperately wanted to work with a team so they could show me their new tricks, just as I had showed others when I was on the street.

For that first ride, I worked with a Crew Chief named Jason, He was one of the most patient teachers I had ever met. I think he actually knew just how scared I was, and instead of "making fun of the boss" (believe me, it would have been easy), he was gentle with me, to make sure I understood what was happening.

That's what I realized – that my Managers were scared as well.

After all, they had not been on the street in years. Although a few of my Managers respond to calls on a normal basis, many times getting there in advance of the unit, others did not. It could have been by coincidence. The point was that we had told everyone who came to work for us that while the life-saving part of our job was certainly what we trained for, it was the "caring" part of EMS that we lived for. That one on one relationship with the patient, holding their hand and telling them that everything would be ok. Frankly, I saw that missing in my Managers.

I also think the customers saw it too. The employees of the company had lost their respect for their Supervisors because they felt they didn't care and couldn't do their job anymore.

You know, EMS is a funny business. Unlike major corporations, where the person promoted is usually <u>never</u>

242

asked to go on the line again, EMS personnel must know that their leaders not only know their job, they must be able to do it. Not some of it, but all of it. And, they must be willing to do so, especially in a pinch.

Some of my own Managers had let me down. I was sure they would want to try this to see if they could improve morale or, at a minimum, get back in touch with their own employees (their customers).

So, we ended this meeting with a request from me; those who wanted to could ride one, 12 hour shift per month, their choice of stations, at their own comfort level. That meant they could even ride as a third person.

Two immediately thought it would not only be fun to get "back in the saddle," but they were excited. Yes, they were probably scared like I was, but like me, never showed it. Those two Managers rode on Ambulances for the next few years when they could. They made me proud.

In the meantime, I still wait to see who else will jump *back on the horse.*

I'm not mad at them. In fact, I feel a little sorry for them.

Most are simply just afraid.

Trauma Dave

I would like to think that, as a Paramedic, I have helped a great number of people get into this business. Most came to me as a student, and I watched them blossom into a good, and sometimes GREAT practitioner.

This story is about one of those great ones. David was very young when he first came to us (one of the youngest – around 18), but what he lacked in age, he more than made up for in ambition, intelligence and the passion we all feel when we are treating our patients.

David was assigned to unit 410 as a Paramedic student. In regards to that assignment, I must tell you that most students don't sign up for this unit because we were busy – VERY busy. Some thought it was just "too much work." This unit was commonly referred to as "the trauma unit." We were also known as "the night unit." What that meant is that most shifts began very quietly (we checked the truck and went to sleep, all before 9 AM), knowing that 3 or 4 PM rolled around, we would be toned out for our first of many calls. From that point, we would rarely see the station for the remaining 16 hours (we worked a 24 hour shift at the time, so we worked 7 AM to 7 AM).

The other name had more to do with the unit's location than anything else. The location of 410's station ended up to be a prime location if you wanted to learn about trauma. With two major interstate highways and two major State roads running through our district, not to mention the various bars and hang-outs for potential/future patients, the area was ripe to see everything you needed to see to become a seasoned trauma veteran. What was interesting is that one of the interstate highways was still being built and not open for business yet. Even with that, we found ourselves driving onto the yet-unopened road to find our fair share of cars, usually upside down, usually driven by drunken somebodies who either didn't know the interstate wasn't open yet or knew that it wasn't and, therefore, a place they could drive even FASTER than the normal highway.

Our station was so close to where the two major State highways met that we had an area kindly known as the "knife and gun club" arenas of the County.

So, in conclusion, If you wanted to get trauma training, we were it!

From the day Dave first appeared at our station, we knew he was different, in three distinct ways. First, not satisfied with checking off the truck and watching TV, he wanted to know what everything was, what it all did, how he could use it to help people. He wanted to know if he could touch, put together, test or whatever – he was truly interested in learning everything about his craft.

The second way he was different was the way he stood up and took control of a patient's condition. Many students like to sit back and wait for us to tell them to do something, but not David. He was protective of our patients, while giving a genuine caring for their condition and wanting to make things better. He was a definite caregiver and that would carry him for many years.

The third difference was not exactly a positive one, nor was it a negative. It was simply something everyone had to know if he was to be a student on your unit.

Most Paramedic students carry a sort of "white cloud" with them, which many crews like. When these students come to ride, it gets very quiet and calm. No bleeding stumps, no decapitations, no shootings, and no head-on car crashes.....nothing! It's not good for the student (they have to have patients to get their credits and their teaching moments are made when people get sick or injured) but, in a way, it's great for the patients – and the crews who can always stand a rest.

Unfortunately, there was a different cloud around David, hence his loving nickname given to him by my partner and I, "Trauma Dave."

We knew from the moment he got on the truck (ok, probably the 2nd shift) that every time he worked, we could expect the end of the world! Spectacular car crashes, multiple shooting, stabbings, patients with severe lacerations or life-threatening bleeders, all came out to play when Dave was on board.

To say that he got his "teeth cut" at 410, was a slight misrepresentation of the facts. We ALL got our trauma expertise when he was working with us. David saw more trauma (and helped more people and learned more things) than any student we ever had.

But, as I have said before, there was something else. David also had more passion, more "common sense" (I know I shouldn't use the "C" word, but let's face it, it's a disappearing process) and more "gumption" than anyone I knew. He always had a smile, always was positive on any given situation and always, ALWAYS put the patient first.

That's not to say that all students didn't have that view. Many students, I think, felt intimidated having two seasoned veterans on the unit and not wanting to make them angry by asking a question. For the record, Tim and I NEVER got mad at a student for any question, but I guess there were a few who did. So, usually, they would stand in the corner and watch, waiting for us to ask them to do something.

I could never understand that thought process, so that is probably why I was a big pain to those of the profession who mentored me. I constantly asked questions about treatment, equipment, diseases, *what was that REALLY* and other things I wanted to know about. Dave had that same quality.

In all fairness, I also realized that many students held a full time job (24 hours on and 48 off) while going to school. I remember those days in which you would work your 24, get off at 7 AM, travel to class for 10 hours, study either at the library or at home (with all of those life issues getting in the way of school), wake up early the next day to either spend a full day at the Hospital or doing ride time (both usually going into night hours), rush home for 4-5 hours of sleep and, then, back to work for another 24 hour shift. I understood if they were tired.

Having said that, I also didn't have much sympathy for them. All of the students were told of the grueling schedule and all embraced it. If you had a passion for this job, you would simply make it happen. Your family generally jumped on board with you, supporting your decision and knowing, at least for that 9 month period, that your life was not your own. The idea that we should all get 8-10 hours of sleep every night is, we all know, a dream. In this job, you're lucky if you get 6 (when you're off duty). School, family, children's activities and all that is in between in our normal lives become compounded when you are trying to ride a minimum of 1,000 hours, see patients in the Hospital, study for the next exam and keep your sanity.

Passion – that is really what it's all about.

I am proud to say that David went on to teach many Paramedics, just as we taught him. And, I found out later, he never forgot. Some 20 years later, he was a highly regarded Physician assistant in a large trauma center.

We met some years later at an EMS conference where we were both speaking. I had been on the speaking circuit for some time so I introduced Dave to everyone that I knew. He was a tremendous teacher and I wanted to see if I could get him into this circuit.

As I introduced him to a friend, I mentioned he had been a student and now a PA and he went out of his way to tell my friend that I had "taught him everything I knew about trauma and Paramedicine."

I have to admit that stopped me for a moment. I was proud and awed he would even remember all of that. Yes, I know he was studying and learning, but honestly, we were just imparting what we knew so it would help him. As he continued to tell my friend about 410 and the trauma he saw, he made me very proud. Here he was, a Physician's Assistant, surpassing his teacher in knowledge and experience – and yet, he was thanking me for starting him out.

I truly didn't know what to say. But, I do now.

Dave, when you read this, remember that you were the most talented of all my students. Tim and I were constantly amazed by your knowledge, your questions (yes, we had to look a lot of them up), your passion for always doing the right thing and your ability to "think on your feet" as a student and, later, as a Senior Crew Chief and PA.

Dave has had a tremendous career as a Paramedic, a Nurse and a Physician Assistant. For all of his patients, I hope they understand how lucky they are to have him as their caregiver.

Thanks, Dave. You are the best – and you make me proud every day!

The Email

It came in on a Friday afternoon.

The fact that it was April 1st made me a little suspicious, but there was no denying it. Cliff's name was on it. I realized it wasn't a joke.

It was one of those automatic emails we all put up when we are going to be out of town. "I'm out of the office until February 8, 2010. I am currently deployed with the US Dept. of Health and Human Services, Disaster Medical Assistance Team SC-1."

The problem was (among other things) was that I received the email on Friday, April 1, 2011, one year after those dates.

The larger problem was, of course, was that the person who had sent it, Cliff Parker, had died one year and a week before I received his simple but shocking email.

Cliff continued to teach us, even as he had left early.

When a co-worker dies, there are many things those who are left must do to keep an organization (or family) going. Mourning, of course, is primary, but operationally, there are many things you wouldn't even think of. Over the days following his death, I dialed his office number, just to hear his voice mail message. When do you take that off? When do you delete his e-mail address? What things does HR need for his widow? What about his office? What about the service?

And, now - we know - what was his email account?

Of course we had his phone forwarded to someone in the office and, eventually, recorded the voice mail message (to hear later) so we could get that changed. Now, one year later, I had to talk with the computer folks about getting his vacation request off of the email system. There's not a person who is reading this who hasn't forgotten to turn their vacation message off after returning to work (that's why friends remind us when we get back, to take it off).

I guess Cliff never did – because he got so sick when he came back.

And, a vacation, it was not. As an Executive Officer for the South Carolina DMAT (Disaster Medical Assistance Team), he slept in trucks, on the ground and, most of the time, simply didn't sleep at all, taking care of the thousands of people left homeless in various disasters, this most recent one in Haiti.

I asked him several times over the next six weeks following his diagnosis of pancreatic cancer how the people of Haiti were – you hear the stories and read the papers but you don't know if that is the truth or not. Cliff, in his wonderful self, told me of gracious people who were very glad that the Americans were there and very kind to everyone they met.

This is the guy I lived through Katrina with. While craziness was going on around him, all he could think about is how kind people were. I have to admit they were kind. When you were around Cliff, everyone seemed to be kind.

I sit reading his email over and over. A friend who received this same e-mail mentioned to me how sad it was to receive and how much they missed him.

It all happened so fast. Cliff had just returned from Haiti when he got sick and went to the Hospital the following day. From that point on, he was in a battle for his life. At the young age of 50, we never imagined we would be burying him six weeks later. He lost his battle with pancreatic cancer on April 25, 2010.

We had just buried our wonderful former EMS Director, Ray Graham, about 9 months earlier. He was held in very high regard. Ray had cancer as well, however, he had beaten it once, living an extra few years before it took him. He had started the service that was to be recognized as the one everyone else in the State went to when they had a question. His heritage continues today.

Cliff was, at first, a Paramedic and, eventually, a Senior Crew Chief with our system. He left to be an Assistant Director with a rural service. When I took over as Director in Charleston, we had an opening for a safety Officer and Cliff was perfect for it. In his former job, he would drive

40 miles every day to work. His work with us would put him less than 10 miles from his office. It wasn't a hard sell and I will be forever grateful that he decided to come home.

Now, I stare at the email again.

"I am out of the office…..." How could we have missed this? I know that no one sent emails after he had died but they had to see it when they sent a "get well" email while he was sick.

It doesn't matter. It's there.

Then, I remember something else. April 1st is more than April fool's Day. It is also Ray Graham's birthday and he is a King of tricksters! I wonder if he and Cliff are somewhere in heaven, hunched over a computer (a heavenly one, of course. It never freezes, always works and NEVER has to be rebooted). Cliff wants to send this but knows it might distress some. Ray elbows him and winks.

At first, the e-mail makes me very sad. As I think through it, I get a small smile on my face and realize that Cliff is trying to tell me something.

When he was very sick and the time was near, I told him when he got to the other side, he could send me the winning lottery numbers and I would be fine with that. He smiled, too weak to talk.

Instead, I reread the e-mail again, and again.

"I'm out of the office….."

Cliff, you always made people laugh and you always put us at ease.

Thanks for the note to let us know you're ok.

We miss you.

Best Friends

We have all had best friends; most are from our childhood.

At this writing, I am at the fourth day of a four-day weekend with one of my closest friends. I have come to be with my friend who is in the Hospital.

I realize that many just don't have that type of time to take off of work and life to go to a Hospital room and sit with your friend.

My retort to that? – I'll tell you at the end.

But, I digress.

Neal is one of those long-time friends, someone I have known since the 5th grade.

There are many friends we have, most of which have faded in and out of our lives, either due to moving or other situations that come before us during this adventure we call life. We all hate when that happens, but it is inevitable in most cases.

However, if you think about it, there are a few friends in our lives who have stayed the test of time. Neal is one of those. He and I have been linked by our lives in Junior and Senior High School, adventures in life and, generally, just being good friends.

We are an unlikely friendship. Anyone who is familiar with life in High School will understand what I am about to describe.

Neal was a member of the "fat-kids" group. I am not using that word in a derogatory manner, but by which it was used in High School (yes, I know it was used derogatorily there as well but if you remember, it was also used as an identifier). So that you don't think I would ever leave myself out of this, I was in the "skinny-kids-that-get-their-butt-kicked-daily" group. Neal was a Photographer, something that in High School, I knew nothing about. I was a chorus kid, someone with an OK voice but a terrible defensive posture.

Neither Neal, nor I went out for any type of sports. Neal instead, overwhelmed himself with the photography side, buying cameras that were very expensive but very good. He became the lead Photographer for the yearbook.

Everyone knew Neal. They didn't want to be "friends" with him (again, those knowing the High School culture) but they were always nice – when they wanted their picture in the school newspaper or yearbook. At all other times, it was as if he didn't exist.

Neal however, would have none of it. On top of his talent for photography, Neal also read everything he could get his hands on. Some things that the school wouldn't like (we called them subversive in those days) were his favorites. He knew way more than most of us at that age and had the ability to "discuss" (some of us would call argue) the finer points of almost anything. He was one of the most learned people I knew.

I think the main reason many kids didn't like him was jealousy. They knew he had much more knowledge than they did and that scared the hell out of them. Standing back, it was an interesting thing to watch as a friend.

And now, the guy who was probably smarter than most of our teachers, the guy who had a zest for life that only the smallest football player could hope to appreciate – that guy was losing the final battle. And a battle it was.

About 5 years after having beaten kidney cancer, he called me and said he had lung cancer, stating it as calmly as if he was telling me he was going to go to the store. This guy, the one who didn't smoke, didn't drink, didn't use recreational drugs (or any other for that matter) was dying.

With five years passed on the first cancer and minus one kidney as a result, he went on with life. We had thought he had truly "beaten the beast." He was "disease free," as he called it, until the point when he found it had returned in his lungs.

At that time, he told me he felt good, he didn't feel sick and he was going to "fight this thing as hard as I can." I cheered him on and told him that a positive attitude was half of the battle. I pledged to be there for him, no matter what he needed.

What I didn't know at the time, but we found out in the next few weeks, was that the cancer he was talking about was an "aggressive" form, one that would quickly form in his head in the form of 4 brain tumors, in his left hip (near where they took his kidney) and the liver. That last one we found out about when I arrived here shortly after he called to tell me the news of his returned cancer.

I flew in on a Friday and met with the Hospice Nurse. The local Hospice, according to Neal, had just told him he couldn't come on board but all of that was just a mistake. I finally saw Neal that Friday night.

The minute I entered the room, many of the tools that I had used in my years as a Paramedic, returned. I looked across the room at the friend who had stuck with me no matter what, had always been honest with me and had never wavered in his love for me like a brother, lying asleep in the bed. He looked a tinge of yellow. My senses told me he had only days left.

Saturday came and I got there shortly after breakfast. To say that his drug level was a little elevated was to say the least. Although Neal could see me and eventually realize who it was, everything else appeared to be in a difficult order. He continued to have a conversation in that "slurred drugeeze" language you hear, mostly just before they put someone under for major surgery.

I am sure he had a great talk with me – although I didn't understand what he was saying and he probably never remembered our conversation – but we were together – and that was important to both of us.

I returned after lunch to find Neal much more awake and verbal. I spent most of the afternoon, talking about everything and about nothing – mostly about friendship stuff, reliving the past.

It was obvious after that talk that Neal was in deep denial.

I had thought that was the case when we talked on the phone two weeks before. He had mentioned that he had just come out of the Hospital and that he was going for another treatment in a few weeks. I asked him why.

"Well….." he said.

Then - nothing. It was obvious he hadn't thought that through. But, that wasn't true. He had actually thought it through well but just hadn't gotten the answer he wanted.

I told him not to answer that question right now but to think about why he wanted to go through another round of treatment and that we would talk the following Sunday.

When I talked to him that Sunday, I asked him again if he had thought about the question. He said he had and that the answer was that he wanted to do it if he could get maybe two or three weeks - and then he stopped. He started to cry.

That was the conversation that drove me to drop everything and be with my friend. I realized that I had to come down and see my friend, to touch his hand, to see his face. As I said, it's hard to tell how sick someone is over the phone. I didn't know what I could do, but at the beginning of this battle, I had told him I would fight right alongside of him, with one caveat; when it was time, I was going to tell him and he had to listen.

When people sign onto Hospice, those wonderful people do what they do best. They help people to be comfortable in their final days and hours. If Neal were to sign on to Hospice and, suddenly, want to sign off to *get* treatment, that meant that much of Hospice's long standing treatments could not be done. It was the equivalent of setting about to fix an engine but realizing you would never get the right parts. You continued to use 2 days' time to fix the engine and then, suddenly, you stop and take some of the engine apart.

I don't know if that makes any sense, but that is how Hospice works. You sign on and they have the plan. If you want to fight, you don't sign on. It's as simple as that.

It was apparent that the time had come to have that discussion with him. This is the discussion about time being short. I had spoken to hundreds of patients in the back of the Ambulance, being truthful with them when I thought it might be time.

Don't get me wrong. I fought for every patient I had – but they also demanded someone to be truthful with them. Most had been in Hospitals and had been given that *don't worry – everything is going to be ok* look from Nurses when they knew that wasn't true.

Neal started to get tired and I told him to go ahead and get some sleep. I would go and eat dinner and be back with him Sunday. I left him with his girlfriend Vickie, at his side.

Sunday came and I got to the room around 1 PM. Neal was doing well, although sleeping more than normal. Vickie and I left him for a minute and walked to the snack room.

"He isn't going to leave the Hospital," she said matter-of-factly.

"No, I don't believe he is," I confirmed.

She looked troubled. "Really?" It was then I realized that although she had been a wonderful companion to this man for over 10 years, he had almost sold her on the *don't worry, sweetie, I'll be home soon* view, while he fought the disease.

"I don't think he has 30 days left," I said. We continued to talk about converting the bed to a Hospice bed so he could stay there and be comfortable. The Hospital was in with that and it seemed it would be the best course of action for him.

We returned and the cooking channel was on. Neal was looking at the show, as if he was as sharp as ever. When he opened his mouth, it was a little slurred but he started to talk about the wonderful things they made on this channel and I should start watching the Iron Chief because it was so good.

I went over to the edge of his bed and sat next to him. I told him we had to have a talk.

Calmly, he asked Vickie if she could leave us alone for a minute and she left. I asked Neal if he knew where he was and what day it was (he looked at me curiously but realized I was trying to find out how clear he was).

I asked him if he remembered our agreement on the fight. He asked if I meant "the talk?" and I shook my head in agreement.

"Yes," he said. "I remember."

And, it was then that I started to explain to him that this was it and I thought we were pretty close to the end of the race. Neal got very serious and listened very closely.

At the end, he looked at me and said, "So, you don't think I should go through with the other treatments?" I told him no. I knew in my mind that he would never live two weeks to see another treatment but felt I needed to be as honest as I could with him. I had promised him I would.

We both looked down, the way men do when they don't want to talk about something sensitive, and both looked back at one another. He started to cry again.

All I could do at that moment is to lean over and hold his head in my chest. I told him that he had been the bravest patient I had ever seen and that he had fought a good fight. He mumbled, "This is so hard. I just don't want to suffer like my Mom did."

I remembered his mother's long illness years before and how pain management had improved.

We straightened up and I told him that this WAS hard – and he was doing such a good job. With that, we both said goodbye and I mentioned that I would see him today just before I left to go home.

As I left the room, I spoke with Vickie and told her I thought we had a good discussion and that he was more accepting of what was to come. We hugged and I left to go back to the hotel.

I don't think I had ever been as tired as I was then.

The following day, I came in around noon and found Neal awake but somewhat groggy. He said they had just given him his pain medication and he was sleepy. I told him to take a snooze and I would wait here. He slept.

Except for the rude therapy dog woman (yes, I know the animals are supposed to be good for patients, but, cripes, he was SLEEPING!), he had a peaceful afternoon. He awoke around 4 PM and we discussed what we had talked about the other day. He understood.

Two friends entered and he and I said our goodbyes.

I drove to the airport and came home.

AFTERNOTE: Neal died peacefully in his sleep nine days after I left. One of the discussions we had in the room dealt with his inability to see Christ as his Savior. As a good Christian, I know I should have spent some time going over that and "showing him the way," but, I didn't. I knew Neal well enough to know that he wasn't really an atheist but probably an agnostic. I did mention that one of us was going to be right – and if it was me, he owed me a steak dinner when I got there.

"How do you know you're going to make it?" he asked with a smile.

"I guess we'll just have to see," and we both laughed.

I know I had mentioned at the beginning on the issue of not being able to take off of work and life to go to a Hospital room and sit with your friend.

Let me make it clear; when a dear friend dies, many of us take time out of our busy day to go to the funeral. We look in the box and mention how they either do or don't look natural. The problem is that our friends may have needed us before then. Think of that next time a friend calls you in trouble. Your fancy house, boat, car, etc. are only things and most of them will rust out and be unusable long before your friendships end.

I don't know about you but I plan on having that steak dinner with him one day.

Call the one you love NOW – Don't Wait

It arrived on a Thursday afternoon.

As I pulled the mail out of the box, I noticed the envelope was larger than the rest. It was in one of those business-type manila envelopes but had a hand-written address on it.

Addressed to me, it was from Kip, my friend, Steve's, step-brother.

I didn't understand, though, why Kip would be writing me. When we received the Christmas card back two years ago with a new address on it (forward to Ft. Lauderdale), we assumed Steve had gone home to take care of his Mom. My mom had died early but I often wondered what it would be like to be a 45 year old, returning home to take care of my parents.

I opened it to find our Christmas card from last year, unopened, and a note;

Dear Don;

Thank you for keeping in touch with Steve for all of these years. I'm sorry to have to tell you that Steve died of a heart attack last year. I have a tape of Mary Plus Three which I still listen to. It makes me smile. Take care of yourself. Sincerely, Kip.

Steve, I and two other friends, Len and Mary, had been together as a singing group, *Mary Plus Three*.

We had started in 1968, formed in those strange years of High School. I don't remember exactly how we got started, but I knew we were challenged by someone to perform in front of someone besides students. Steve and Mary had been friends before I had met either one of them, although I knew both. They were fantastic talents, whose voices one day were sure to be famous. I had wished on several occasions that I had a voice as talented as Steve's.

They asked me to join the group and soon, Len joined, a great bass voice and talented guitar player. Together, we called ourselves *Mary Plus Three*. Mary, Len and I played guitar. Steve played most of our percussion - a tambourine, and sang.

During that time, we kidded that we ought to change the name. Various ideas came up from *Three Kings and the Girl* (our favorite) to *Three Thorns and a Rose* (Mary's favorite). None the less, we remained *Mary Plus Three* and became very close friends.

Our first engagement was the Women's Group of the Plantation Golf Club. We thought that would be it, but soon found ourselves traveling all over the City of Ft. Lauderdale and Miami, singing for whoever wanted to hear us - Church groups, bowling leagues and even a stint at the Four Seasons in Miami. We practiced every

Saturday at Mary's house (her parents were <u>so</u> strict) and tried to remember our music. We did not have any way of recording the group as the smallest recorder stood 7 feet tall and required six men to move (not to mention the cost of buying one).

We ended up making a record (a collector's item to this day as we sold all 100 of them), traveled to Washington, DC, and singing in the National Cathedral and the Kennedy Center. We also toured Central America. We loved what we were doing and enjoyed making new sounds. It was a magical time in our lives.

. . . .

In all of my years, as a person and a Paramedic, nothing hit me as unfair as the note. How could someone so talented, so full of life, be dead? He was younger than me, 47, and looked like he did from his High School days. He was one of those friends who seemed to never age (except for the beard).

And, just like that, he was dead. *A heart attack. How could that be? He ate very healthy, exercised, always had a positive attitude.* God had made a mistake.

I remember sitting up in my bedroom, crying and screaming that it was wrong, that it couldn't be. My wife stood beside cradling my head. I felt so lost.

. . . .

In 1988, we had reunited (after 17 years) to sing again. We met at Mary's parent's house, now in another city than the one we grew up in. It was the first time we had been together since graduation. I remember Steve arriving by motorcycle and the fact that he looked like he had never changed made me a little jealous.

Sure, he had the beard, but he looked as young and vibrant as ever. His voice was very strong and wonderful as I remembered. We sang, not remembering much of the words but certainly remembering the warmth our music gave to each other.

At that time, we decided we would get together for our music teacher's retirement party, set for that coming June. We met in Ft. Lauderdale at a restaurant and sang for the woman who had started it all. Many have a teacher who changed their lives while in school. Ms. McNamara was that teacher for us. She taught us all that you could do whatever you put your mind to. As a surprise, we sang for her and she cried. I think we all did that night.

Later in the year, we decided that getting together was fun. Although Steve lived in California, he came home (Florida) to visit family and, since the rest of us lived in Florida at the time, it would not be that hard to get together and sing for - whom? Well, Mary was a music teacher, so we could certainly sing for those kids. Then, we thought of all the children who would be in Hospitals during Christmas and decided to see if we could sing for them.

It was a natural fit. Children are very honest about music (they either like it or hate it but won't sugar coat their opinion) and we enjoyed making their lives a little more bearable in a time, that was probably pretty low for them.

The last time we were together was December of 1988. We did a rather heavy tour session and realized we were very tired and it was starting not to be fun. Sticking to our guns (if it stops being fun, we should stop for a while), we bid goodbye to everyone as we went back to our lives, knowing that we would all live well into our 90's and still be able to get together and reminisce.

……………..

It seemed so strange, the envelope in my hands. Kip was Steve's younger brother (½ brother actually) and, I found out later, had gone on to medicine as a PA. Steve spoke of him whenever we asked about his family. You could tell that as a step brother, he was a step brother - but Steve admired him as someone who had done well in his life.

Having a brother myself, I watched many of my friends fight with their siblings. One close friend had literally fistfights with his brother, calling him names that were both angry and hurtful. I was very glad my brother and I had been as close as we had. I don't think either one of us have ever said a bad word about each other at any time in our lives. I consider my brother my closest friend, a father figure in my life. I love him so much and consistently tell people that I had better be the first one to die as I couldn't stand living if he weren't around. Although I smile when I say that, I am deeply serious about it.

I brought the envelope into the house and noted to my wife that the address was the one we had sent Steve's Christmas card this year. Although he lived in California, we managed to talk at least once a year, usually after he received our card. With the time difference, I stopped calling him (too early) and he would call me (a mutual agreement) and we would catch up on old times. He had bought a piece of land there and was earning money as a restaurant Manager trying to buy another one. Quite the entrepreneur he was.

This note hit me as hard as anything I had ever read.

Steve, the one who looked as young as he had in High School, the no-meat, non-smoker, healthy eating kind of guy - was dead of an MI.

I guess a lot of things went through my mind at that moment. The first was that Steve, while still hundreds of miles away, had been one of my closest friends in High School and I considered him a close friend even today. He was a guy who should have been hanging out with all of the cool kids but didn't mind a skinny dweeb who wasn't on any sports team, hanging with him. When the skinny dweeb hit a wrong note or pronounced words wrong, he didn't laugh at me - he laughed with me. He had a deep smile that always told you he was your friend, in the best and worst of times. He was that friend that would stand up to those cruel kids we all knew in High School and tell them "bite me" when they would make fun of the skinny kid.

Since I had a father that drank more than most fish, I would move from friend to friend for the weekend, spending the night there instead of enduring another night of his noisy clamoring of why we all weren't going to bed at six like we should. While I sometimes felt like I was somewhat of a burden at some houses (after all, I ate there as much as their own children), Steve understood and never made me feel unwelcome.

And, now, he was dead. A year ago! I can't believe it.

We have friends whom we have managed to stay in touch with, although they are rare in our lives. Instead, we write Christmas cards and have occasional telephone calls to see "what's up." Steve lived in California, which made conversation even harder with the time change.

Yeah, I know. They are all excuses. The simple truth is that we lose touch with time. We forget our friends and move through our lives. We don't mean to. We just do.

Even though it had been a year since I had talked with Steve, he was such a good friend; he still lived in my heart. And, now, I was sadder than I had ever been before.

Of the four of us, Steve was probably the healthiest. I don't mean to say that he didn't have his fair share of partying, but the last time we talked, he was a vegetarian, didn't smoke, drank only wine and looked *just like he did in High School.* To those of us who had put on a few pounds since then, we were jealous.

He also sang just as beautiful as he had during those years. A beautiful tenor voice, he had passion when he sang. He honestly enjoyed it, even when it was hard.

I suppose this is so hard for me because Steve is the first close friend who has died in my life. On top of that, I found out a year later than when it happened. I have had an unofficial Uncle die about one year before I found out. The delay in that case was due to his wife (my unofficial Aunt, of course) who couldn't call me due to her own devastation. I understand that, in a way, and yet, I was still mad.

People say that grieving is done in everyone's own time, but I know from experience that grieving a year after the fact hurts even worse. You want to be there for your friend, and would, no matter what time of day or night they called, no matter where they lived and no matter what situation they were in. You *assume* that you will be there when they die, to offer support to their family and friends.

However, in this case, there is none of that. Only a one page letter written by one of my best friend's brother that he is dead.

The following day, while driving to work, I imagined what I would have said to him now, if he were able to hear me (and who knows what you are able to hear after you're gone. For all I know, he was sitting right next to me).

"Steve," I would have started. "You meant so much to me in my life. I will never forget your friendship, your brotherly way you helped me, you protected me and you respected me. You made those last years in High School bearable. You laughed at my stupid jokes, never made fun of my clothes and always had feelings for me and my thick glasses (as you had yours, too)."

"I have an older brother," I would tell him. "But, I have always considered you my younger brother as well. Thank you for your caring and your friendship. I will miss you."

So, I have said it. Here, for you to read (and maybe him while he is sitting in the heavenly library - or wherever).

If you have a friend whom, while you are reading this, you are reminded of them and remember that you haven't talked to them in a while - maybe a long while - do yourself a favor. Put this book down, go to the telephone (not the computer!) and give that friend a call. Tell them how much you mean to them and then chat for a bit.

Maybe about important stuff, possibly about silly stuff. It really doesn't matter.

Call them now. Put this book down and do it. You won't regret it. You never know what's going to be around time's corner.

Tim

As I sit in the small dining room of a non-descript assisted living facility in North Carolina, I feel bad for my friend, Tim, my former EMS partner, whose mother had recently died. I was there to honor her, although we had never met. I was actually there for my friend, my partner, who most likely felt lost and alone. I know I did when my mom died.

…………….

Just 40 years ago, I started my career in EMS, skinny, shiny and new with green around my ears (or so the old guys told me) and ready to save the world.

Six years later, I am to meet Tim, my partner, and as this book is written, still the longest standing partnership in our EMS company's history (that may be because they disbanded the organization when another Public Safety entity took it over, but we'll take whatever we can get).

The time with Tim, was special for me. I remember the first day we met, out at station 410, also called the "trauma unit" (also called *The Buffalo Roadhouse*). He had not seen much trauma (i.e., ANY) and was looking forward to working in that arena.

Over the next 5 years, we would work together, putting people back together, counseling those who thought the end was near (or those who wanted to end it sooner), assisting those who could not breath, delivering a patient's fifth baby (no first baby is ever delivered quickly) and, in most cases, holding the hand of those who thought they were dying. Many were not, but it was the worst time in their lives and we were the ones holding them together.

Tim was, by far, the best partner I ever had. That's hard to say, considering the Veterans I had worked with. Lee was, of course, my "EMS daddy", the one who taught me everything. There was Becky, the one who I originally hated, because I thought she had taken my slot when they were hiring, only to learn later that she and I were in the same boat (the company didn't want either one of us on the street – me because of my dispatching skill, her because she was a woman).

Tim and I went through a lot together and continue to be close friends. That seems strange, because we were not close friends while we worked together. That is, in my opinion, why we were such great partners.

. . . .

The service for Tim's Mom starts. Tim tells everyone that he was going to read something but he felt that he couldn't now and would probably start crying. I leaned to my wife Barbara and reminded her that I would not make her read anything at my funeral if she promised that I didn't have to read anything at hers.

He asked a friend to start the service with a prayer and then there was music.

We had both seen people become closer friends while they worked together and the disastrous situations that caused. When a mistake happened (yes, there are mistakes just like anywhere else), it was difficult for those who were *friends* to be honest to their partners about it. That was not a problem for Tim and me.

In fact, I can honestly say he saved my career – and my life one night.

It was somewhat of a typical call. A 70-something male was having trouble breathing and, in my estimation, he was in CHF (Congestive Heart Failure). We knew the treatment for it. Oxygen, IV access, 40 mg of Lasix (the medicine that makes you pee) to relieve the fluid and support them to the Hospital.

Things were going well, the oxygen was helping him, however, I could not get an IV on the patient. We were well into transport and after three attempts, I decided not to cause him pain any further since the oxygen was helping him.

We arrived at the ER and turned the patient over to them. Tim and I returned to the unit, cleaned it up, finished our report and headed back to the station.

It was unusually quiet, that drive back to 410. Tim turned to me.

"Do you think that guy had CHF?" he asked.

"Yeah," I said. "Didn't he?" Now I was asking myself, instead of being sure and that somewhat bothered me.

"No, I don't think so," he said, looking a little perturbed.

Now, it was not unusual for us to disagree about what the issue may be – not many times but it certainly happened on occasion. Usually, one of us would follow up the next shift to find out who was closer to what we thought the issue was.

Tim looked rather upset with this one and it didn't seem like we were going to settle this quickly.

He started to discuss the various vitals and hints that we both saw and, I realized, he was right. This patient had emphysema and he was having an attack.

What's the difference between CHF and Emphysema? Congestive Heart failure is when, for a variety of reasons, you have too much fluid for your heart (or in some cases, normal fluid but your heart is unable to pump it due to damage). The primary thought regarding treatment of these patients is to decrease the load of fluid, usually through diuretics which are medications which allow the body to dump fluid through urination.

Emphysema, on the other hand, is a lung disease, caused by different things, however, the primary issue is that your body can't push Carbon dioxide out of the system (after breathing in oxygen and exchanging gases) and, because of that, the body becomes unbalanced in their acid/base balance (PH). They are usually already dehydrated.

"It's a good thing you didn't give him the Lasix," he said. "You would have really hurt him."

It was then that I realized he was absolutely right and that I had made a mistake.

Now, for those reading this who are Paramedics and EMTs, we all must admit that making a mistake is a big ego downer. We pride ourselves on being *on the mark* on what we do, and our pride makes us believe we really rarely make mistakes.

"How much reading do you do?" Tim asked, now obviously ticked.

"I read," I indignantly told him.

I had just read the newspaper that morning and did everything I can to be abreast of current events – and, of course, the comic page.

"I mean articles, textbooks, medical things," he now said, confirming what I was thinking.

How did he know what I was thinking?

We didn't talk much as we went back to the station that night. He was mad that such an obvious patient had slipped through my hands – and so was I.

As the music ended, several people got up to talk about Tim's Mom. They mentioned how kind she was and how she would engage anyone in a conversation. They all said they missed her a lot.

Then, Tim got up. He started to talk about her. He mentioned that she was somewhat set in her ways and stubborn – and I realized that I may have met her through Tim.

He was kind to everyone (even the guy who kicked him in the chest) and always wanted to help. He was *set in his ways* when treating a patient, realizing that the treatment should do *that* and that the patient should be compliant so *that* could happen. He got frustrated when a medication didn't work or a procedure was thwarted by a patient.

But, kind he was.

As he talked about his Mom, he started to get choked up. I wanted to go up and stand with him but I didn't want him to feel awkward. We waited and he eventually finished his thought. I think people who can do that are some of the bravest people I know

Tim was one of them.

………

Beyond what I saw at work, I didn't know Tim outside of work for many years. We never socialized, never hung out together when we were off duty, never played cards, hunted, went on drunken binges, shared the same girl, camped out, or anything to reflect the tight partnership we had at work.

I think it was what made it all work so well.

After our discussion that day, long ago, I realized that I really hadn't read any medical journals or gotten any new books. I was really in that *I know everything so why should I need to read about it* thought process, not understanding that medicine changed *daily,* and certainly our treatment changed with every new medication, procedure or disease.

The day following that conversation, I went to the bookstore (a reminder that there was no internet at the time) and bought what I thought would help, as it discussed the differences between CHF and Emphysema and how to find them. I brought it to work the next day.

"Thanks," I told Tim. "You were right. I probably was as lazy as one could be while still having fun at their job. I promise that won't happen again."

I saw Tim smile and then he asked me about the book.

I realized soon after that, that he had probably saved my life – my career – by letting me know that learning never ends in this job.

……………..

At the service closed, Tim pointed out to everyone that she was somewhat of a proper woman, making sure she was dressed properly before going out. During the end, she asked for a large T-shirt she could wear so that visitors wouldn't be so shocked by her loss of weight.

Tim showed the crowd the t-shirt he picked – it was the most hideous shirt he could find – and he placed it on his Mom as a last tribute to her. You'd have to understand Tim and his antics, but I do believe it was a son showing the love for his Mom. By that action, he showed her that he didn't care how she was dressed, how stubborn she might be or what she looked like; he loved her unconditionally.

Isn't that what we want to say to all of our Moms?

As I got up to hug Tim, I realized that through all of that, even as we hadn't been *friends* during our partnership, we were probably closer friends than we ever realized.

Years later, Tim realized that Post Traumatic Stress had crept into his life as a result of the many horrible things he had seen, the patients who he felt should have been saved and weren't and the ever-present *"could I have done more"* thoughts that go through our minds every shift.

Tim, I'm here to tell you that you did more for our patients than you could have ever done. The ones who didn't make it did so because of fate or whatever it was that didn't allow us to do magic.

I always remember, though, those patients who had the magic happen and who are walking around today because of what you and I did with them.

Your Mom was proud. I never met her but I know she was.

And I am too.

Thanks Tim.

Lee

I think everyone in this business remembers their first partner.

In the more modern days of EMS, many systems have a training period, anywhere from two weeks or so to several months. They train Field Training Officers to help new employees become accustomed to their new job. There is orientation training, skills testing, leadership training, safety orientation, drivers training – some systems even have an academy that you are trained in.

Not in 1974.

In the private Ambulance business of that day, profit meant everything and there was no money to train anyone. That would take someone out of position, which could otherwise be transporting a patient (making money for the company). So, you may work as a third person for a day or so, just so you knew where the steering wheel and brake pedal were, how to work the stretcher ("VERY important," my trainer would tell me) and how to open and close the rear door (very embarrassing to have a patient ready to load and not being able to get into your Ambulance). In the worst of cases (super-stupid), no more than three days were spent on orientation and, after arrival, you went out in the street as a 2nd person, working with a partner.

I met Lee even before we became partners. I was a dispatcher and Lee was one of the crew who worked the night unit. In this business, everyone worked 24 hour shifts, however the people who worked nights came in at 10 AM and went to sleep. They awoke around 5, went to get dinner and were placed on the street around 7 PM. At that time, all of the day cars were kept out for a short period, usually during the night surge, and eventually brought in around 10 PM to sleep.

That's right. We had no stations out of the main headquarters. If we ran out of night cars (we had a whopping two night units for a city of 750,000), you were awakened out of headquarters and responded to wherever.

As a night person, Lee was a quiet man, one that it took a lot to make laugh. He took his job very serious but was a very nice person. The thing I remember though, being a dispatcher, is his voice.

Lee was always serious when he spoke to me and his voice – well, I have to admit something to you. As a dispatcher, we assigned "personalities" to voices. It didn't matter who they were, it was *how they sounded*. I know that sounds crazy, but if you were to listen to people's voices all day long without much interaction, you too, would start to give personality traits to them.

For Lee, being serious, we kind of took him as someone who was, shall we say, a little uptight – uppity, so to speak. A little mad, kind of snooty. *Looking down at you* kind of thing.

Of course, he wasn't. However, all of the dispatchers thought he was when he talked and he got that persona from us – that he was always mad.

I was soon to find out how wrong I was.

On the very first day, after being transferred from dispatch to the street, I was told that Lee would be my partner. Going out into the parking lot after punching in felt weird. Dispatchers weren't allowed into that area – it felt free! I knew I had made my mark, I was on my way, I was....

"Hey, Lundy!" I heard. I looked over to the unit parked beside the oak tree. "Come on, we haven't got all day."

Lee was a seasoned veteran, some say almost a Doctor. He had a lot of knowledge and I was eager to learn.

"Morning," I said with my big smile and positive voice.

He smiled. I realized I had never seen him smile. "We need to take this unit apart and clean it," he told me, without looking at me. "This unit is FILTHY."

With that, my career started. For the next two hours, we took the entire unit apart, taking bandages out of cabinets, equipment out of holders, cleaning it all and, at the direction of my partner, laying it out on a sheet.

What a waste, I thought. We could just put this stuff back inside. Why is he wasting my time and this perfectly good sheet? We should be out saving lives!

I also noticed that my partner wasn't around for much of the cleaning. He had "stuff" to do and disappeared into the supply shed – or somewhere else. Determined to not let his negativity (as I read it) or his snootiness (as I had heard earlier in my radio days) get to me, I hummed to myself as I gave the equipment the best darned cleaning it had ever seen.

About two hours after we (or I) had started, Lee came out of nowhere and stood by me as I was finishing the last piece of equipment. The Ambulance sat empty.

"Good job," Lee said. Wow, I thought. That's the first positive thing I've ever heard him say. "Now, let's talk learning about each piece of equipment."

Over the next three hours, Lee took me by the hand and individually reviewed with me and taught me about every piece of equipment on that unit. I was not so ego filled to tell myself (or anyone else) that I knew this stuff. I was barely out of EMT school so the only equipment I had seen had been in class. We had spent a whopping 10 hours in the ER looking at sick patients. I hadn't even touched my first patient in need.

Several times, the shift Manager came out and asked what was taking so long. Lee gave him a stern look and told him to go away.

"What is this again?" he would ask. "When would you NOT use this?" he questioned. He gave me the history about much of the equipment that was not taught in class. Tips about their use helped me understand the importance of each piece of lifesaving gear.

"Now, let's put it all back in," he said with a smile. A SMILE! His voice had sounded like he NEVER smiled.

As we put the Ambulance back together, he talked about the positioning of equipment and how I may want some pieces in front of others and the logistics of jump bags and their importance to our work. Most importantly, he talked about what to expect.

As we finished putting the unit together, I realized I wasn't even tired. I was energized. I wanted to go find some sick people!

"I'll be there for you – we're partners," he assured me. "Now, let go eat."

With that, he gave me the keys. I stared at him.

"What?" he smiled again. "You're an Ambulance driver, aren't you? So, drive."

I started to take the keys from him. He pulled them back and squinted at me.

"But don't let anyone call you that," he cautioned. "You're an Emergency Medical Technician. Never forget that."

I don't know if Lee is alive now – we lost touch some years ago. I would have liked to have him read this chapter before it was published.

Lee, if you are out there, thank you. Job well done! I have never forgotten the lessons you taught me at 3419 Nebraska Ave. or the various lessons with our patients. I have never forgotten where I came from or what I am.

Thanks, Lee.

Leadership at Last

I was asleep when the telephone call came.

Barbara, my wife, came in and woke me up with a start. "It's Chief Devine."

I barely opened my eyes, lifted my head, looked at her, and lowered my head back down, reaching for the phone.

"NO, NO," she yelled. "It's Chief Devine. You have to be awake. Get up, get up!"

What was she yelling for? It was like the bed was on fire. I had never seen her like this.

I sat straight up in bed and waivered for a minute. When I thought I was awake, I realized what she was saying. Chief Devine was the Chief that had interviewed me for an EMS Director job just a week ago.

"Hello?" I said into the wired receiver.

"Don?" Chief asked.

"Yes, Chief Devine, great to hear from you," I said as I sat up and tried to sound like I had been awake for hours.

"Don, we've moved down to our finalist and I'd like you to come down to have a talk with me about this EMS Director's job," he said.

I didn't understand.

For months, I had interviewed in every conceivable management position that I could find. Actually, I had even been asked to come to one interview, but all of them were learning situations, some quite frank and others not-so-much.

I had never gotten a call like this.

"That would be great," I said, continuing to sound like someone who didn't want to jump out of his skin and scream. "What about this afternoon?"

Who was I kidding? He was 120 miles away. I realized how desperate it sounded the minute I said it.

The Chief chuckled.

"Well, Don, that's a little soon," he said. "How about next Thursday?"

"Sure," I said, not even knowing if I was working or not. "What time?"

"Let's say 10 AM," he said.

"I'll see you then," I told him.

With that, he hung up and I sat listening to the phone, thinking someone on the other end was going to say, "PSYCH!"

Barbara was standing next to me.

"What did he say?" she asked, almost in a whisper.

"He wants to meet with me," I said.

After all, that is what he wanted, isn't it? He said they had whittled down the candidates and he wanted to meet with me. Then, I thought – how many candidates? Am I one of 50? One of 200?

"What does that mean?" Barbara asked. I decided to find out.

I hit redial and called Chief back. He answered his own phone.

"Chief, this is Don Lundy again," I said as if we were old friends. "Just a question. How many candidates are you meeting with?" I thought it was a fair question and frankly didn't care if it sounded stupid. I needed to know where I stood.

"Just one, Don - you," he said.

Calmly, I looked at Barbara and smiled. "Thank you sir, I'll see you Thursday." I hung up.

I can't really explain how I felt. Excited – scared – no, petrified! My face was on fire – no, my entire body was! I suddenly didn't feel sleepy – in fact, I could have painted the house – TWICE - and then run a marathon with energy left over.

This was it. The Chief wanted to see me – just me – for the EMS Director's job for Hibiscus County.

Next, the worries started to set in.

What in the world did he want to meet with me for? I had completely forgotten that we hadn't talked salary yet and, being that this was the first call back I had ever had, I thought of a hundred things he could be looking for.

As questions went through my mind, I openly shared with my wife about my worries. I discussed the fact that I didn't have a degree and had only a small amount of experience as a leader. I had made mistakes in my first job (who hasn't) but I was sure all of the references would come back golden. Why did he want to see *me*?

Barbara, my wife, has been my rock since we first met at USF in Tampa, Florida. My college roommate, Jim, introduced us. I must say – when we met, it wasn't like bells went off or fireworks happened. However, it did feel – well, natural. It felt as if I had known her for years. We fit so well, thought alike (almost), loved the same things (almost) – she was so pretty and so great and kind and…..well, I digress.

Sitting in our bedroom of the home we had just moved to a year earlier, she sat down next to me and looked me in the eye.

"You're going to do great!" she said, as confident as she always was. "This is what you've been waiting for."

I *have* been waiting for this moment forever. Reading every book I could, moving up through the ranks, obtaining as many instructor certifications as I could and going to several national EMS shows to network with other leaders. I openly went up to leaders I saw, introduced myself and made conversation – or asked them a question. I watched the leaders in our organization learning what to do (and more importantly, what *not* to do).

And, yes, I had waited for this call – and now, here it was.

I don't remember much about the rest of that day – or the rest of that week. Working as a Senior Crew Chief, I had a great job. I took care of patients, all sorts of patients, one patient at a time.

And, now I was driving down to Hibiscus County, population 70,000, mostly retired folks, but a County-wide EMS service with five units.

I don't remember how I got to the front of the Public Safety building, but do remember meeting Chief Devine.

"Don, nice to meet you," he said reaching out his hand.

Chief had been the Fire Chief for the small community until they had made the County-wide service and moved him up to Public Safety Director. They were going to have to hire a fire chef as well.

"So, how much of the town have you seen?" he asked.

"Mostly the main drag but some of the shopping center and the local diner near there," I said.

"Manny's dinner?" he asked. "It's owned locally by a friend of mine. Great place."

He smiled. "Let's go for a ride," he said.

We walked outside to a non-descript car with several antennas and got inside. I noticed he had a car phone in the center of the floor. I admit I was struck! *How progressive is that?* I thought. He could, in fact, drive around within 25 miles of the center of town and talk to anyone by dialing their phone number! The console itself was, of course, Huge!

As we drove, we talked about issues – the employees had sent a letter to unionize and the EMS Directors first projects would be to talk with employees to see if they could be talked out of it. There were some equipment issues and coverage, but the union was obviously on the top of the list.

"So," Chief asked. 'What kind of a leader are you?"

I sat, stunned. No one had ever asked that and, frankly, I had never put it to paper or at least had the thought in my head as to what *kind* of leader I was. I thought telling him that I was the one desperate for this job, would be the wrong message.

"I guess you can say I am a hands-on leader," I stated. "I want to continue to run calls when I can, mix with the troops, learn more about what we do for patients and expand that."

Chief looked at me with a stern look. "Good," was all he said. I wondered if I had given the wrong answer.

We pulled into the parking lot of what I was to learn was the County office building and started towards a large office in the back.

As we entered, the young lady behind the desk said hi to the Chief and to me.

"Is the boss in?" he asked. *The boss* I asked myself. The Chief had a boss?

"Yes and he's expecting you," she answered. He motioned for me to follow him and we entered a large office.

"You must be Don," the large man behind the desk said as he got up and came over to shake my hand. He told me to sit down and it was then I realized he had a couch in his office. Way cool!

"I'm Jimmy Cutwright," he started. "Ron tells me you're our new EMS Director."

Now, my head was starting to spin. I had come down to have a talk with the Chief, we had taken a ride in his phone-laden car and some guy who was the Chief's boss was calling me the EMS Director.

Is this how it's supposed to go? Isn't there an interview (I know I had one before, but I thought this would be like that one, only more detailed).

"Well," I stated. "I sure would like to be."

For the next 20 minutes, we discussed benefits, salary, vehicles, living within the County and various other issues.

Oh, yeah – and the union.

"We can't afford to have a union for the EMS folks," he said. "Do you think you can talk them out of it?"

"Well, I have to be honest," I said. "I was a member of a union at one time and – well, it all depends on why they want one. If we can fix that, we may have a chance."

Both men stared at me without saying a word.

In that brief moment, I thought I had given it all away. *Why did I tell them I was in a union? They won't want me now.*

"Heck, so was I," the Chief chimed in. "But, I came over to the light side."

With that, both men smiled.

"You'll do great," Mr. Cutwright said. "Ron, can you finish up whatever we need?"

Mr. Cutwright shook my hand and said, "Welcome aboard."

The Chief and I exited the office and the woman at the desk wished us a good day. We walked out to his car, got in and he cranked the engine.

As we drove back to his office, he pointed out various points of interest in the city. I didn't even hear what he was saying. I was smiling and nodding, but I had no clue.

He pulled into the parking lot and backed into the space marked, "Chief."

"So," he said. "When can you start?"

Geez, I hadn't even thought of a start day. I could barely speak.

"Let me look at my calendar and see when would be best," I said, trying to sound confident that I could even find my calendar.

"Fair enough," Chief said. "I'll get a letter to you with a proposed salary, a benefit package and a proposed start date. You let me know if that's good or not. We can move it up or back as your schedule permits."

He started to get out of the car and I sat for a minute, unable to move. I then grabbed the handle and opened the door. He had come around to my side of the car by then.

"I think you're going to do great" he said. "See you in a few weeks."

I got back into my car and realized what had just taken place. I had been offered (and evidently accepted), the EMS Directors position for Hibiscus County, Florida.

I don't remember the drive back. I don't remember what I had for dinner that night.

What I do remember is telling the story of the day's events to my sweet wife, who patiently sat at the dinner table and smiled.

Final thoughts and other things that can help you

I have been blessed to be able to be in various places, sitting with various people, many of them extremely talented and smart, while they did a variety of things and dreamed about current issues and the future of this career we call EMS.

At almost every encounter, whether it is with a patient or a meeting about logistics, I always wonder how many lives I have saved, or changed, or even whether I have made a difference at all.

For those whom I have had the honor of meeting – and for the many reading this whom I have not - you *have* made a difference. Some of you are EMTs and Paramedics, others are Law Enforcement Officers, Firefighters, Airplane Builders, Waiters or Waitresses, Janitors, Cooks, Construction Workers – no matter the tool you use to get through the day, believe me, you have made a difference.

You don't think so?

I started in a hearse-type vehicle with a High School diploma, worked my way up the ladder to Supervisor, took a voluntary demotion, got hired as an EMS Director, got fired *without cause*, went back to the field and to school, earning my AS in EMS, then my Bachelor's degree in Health Care (nothing will make you feel young like working full time EMS and attending school with people who could be your son or daughter) and accepted an EMS

Director's position in a fantastic rural system in South Carolina which taught me so much about rural medicine that I continue to use that knowledge every day.

Then, one day, God blessed me with the career choice of a lifetime – to be Director of the Charleston County EMS in Charleston, SC. I call it, "the last bastion of civilization as we know it." It is truly heaven.

That's not bad for a skinny kid from Tampa.

You may be asking yourself, "So what, Don. You may have made a difference, but I still haven't."

Still don't believe me, eh? Follow me here.

Sometime in your life, you may have given advice to someone, talked to somebody about their life habits, their positive attitude or lack thereof, their abilities, their dreams or their fantasies.

For some of you, it's even simpler.

Some of you have sat in a room with a friend, or even maybe someone you barely knew, holding their hand, comforting them - *just by being there.*

Others of you (you know who you are) put $20 in a mailbox for a neighbor who needed some cash to buy groceries. Others went out and mowed someone's lawn that couldn't do it for themselves, for whatever reason – maybe it was just that their lawn mower was broken.

Many of you gave a ride to the Doctor, took a message and delivered it, or maybe it was a simple prayer you said for someone you had met and realized they needed upstairs management's help.

While it's true that you'll never get in the paper for a "hero's" welcome, you may also never know the tremendous difference you made in a person's life.

Believe me, you did.

So, with the future of EMS barreling down the road, what can we, as a career, do to improve our lot in life?

There's so much – and it's so exciting – and, I guarantee – it's hard to do but it is so worth it!

It **is** an exciting time to be in EMS!

Sure, we know the history. In the beginning, we were a group of Funeral Homes doing something that no one else wanted to do. At the time, it was a money-loser, except for the business drummed up when you promised to have your remains handled by the Funeral Home, running the Ambulance you were riding in.

Yes, I know – creepy – but it was what it was. The hearse had the biggest (i.e. fastest) motor of any automobile on the open road at the time, so it served a dual purpose (of which many were glad).

There were some Hospitals which performed Ambulance Services but in some cases, it was an alternate marketing plan. If they took you, you had to go to *their* Hospital.

Private companies, in the beginning, almost all small mom and pops, started in small towns, because no one else would do it. Their neighbors needed them. They managed to make ends meet but never saw any kind of a profit.

One by one, they sold or simply went out of business.

Of course, there were (and are) thousands of Volunteer Ambulance Corps who did it because it helped the community. Some were stand-along agencies and others were Volunteer Fire Departments. The financial plan was barbeque chicken and spaghetti dinners weekly to raise funds to put fuel in the Ambulance (and everything else from oxygen to stretcher sheets). They got up in the middle of the night from a warm bed, in their own home and put on gear to respond to a stranger's house, to help them in their worst medical crisis.

Volunteers, in my opinion, were the true pioneering heroes at the beginning of modern EMS and, in many places in the country, continue to be.

Later, large conglomerate private Ambulance Companies (Wal-Mart sized organizations) started to enter the Ambulance market in droves when they discovered gold (i.e. Medicare) in the transportation of our patients. I don't mean to vilify private services and, if that sounds like what

I am doing, it is far from that. However, I haven't seen any private police forces working a City or County as a for-profit and there is only one for-profit Fire Department that I am aware of.

The reason behind that, is people feel that Law Enforcement and Fire are *essential services*. In time, EMS will be there as well.

When that occurs, for-profit companies will still run Ambulance Services but I think the public will view them quite differently.

Of course, there were others. Some paid Fire Departments attempted to take over private or government EMS services, even the ones which were running well. There were a variety of reasons and many articles and books were written about that subject but the bottom line was that Fire Service, in general, was afraid of losing jobs. They realized (a little late) that they had worked themselves out of a job when they improved construction materials and building standards. Fewer fires, they surmised, meant fewer positions. It made sense at the time.

This is not to say that there aren't tremendous Fire Organizations that do tremendous work in EMS for the right reason. They started EMS in their community from the start and decided that it was going to be done by professionals for the patient, regardless of budget or politics. They have done well since they started and continue to put the sick patient first.

However, as you read this today, there are *merged* Fire/EMS systems that still argue with one another and don't show the best of the best when it comes to patient care. You can discover those services who *took over* another service but who still don't have a clue.

These departments, after *merging,* appear in headlines every day, doing bonehead things that don't put the patient first. They struggle on a daily basis to find identity in the new era of their new department mission of being an EMS service that *occasionally* runs on fire calls.

No matter what you think may happen in the future, I would ask that you never place yourself into the category of those nay-sayers we often here, the "nothing is going to change" gang. Here's why.

Remember, back in the 50's, there was a shocking idea that many said would never work. Technicians, in an Ambulance, that could do what only Doctors could do. They told us that we *may* actually shock a heart in the field!

Many, at the time (the naysayers of that day) said it wouldn't happen. Some were Nurses, others were Physicians, and all feeling it was a crazy idea that wouldn't take hold.

Thank goodness it <u>did</u> happen. In fact, a brave group of Emergency Room Physicians stood up and supported that crazy idea.

There were other *crazy* ideas; An oven that would cook food in a 1/10 of the time, a computer small enough to fit into your home, a portable, battery operated, two-way "walkie-talkie" radio that could transmit beyond 400 feet – heck, they were even talking about telephone you could carry in your pocket.

Crazy? It sure sounded like it then.

However, we know better. The rest is history. Microwave ovens, desktops (now almost obsolete with the Smart phone – a fully operational computer you carry on your belt). Speaking of smart phones, is it just me or are cell phones now used for everything *except* making phone calls?

Paramedics have become the *standard* in field care and now do more for their patient than we could ever imagine.

So, I can try to figure out what is going to happen in EMS for the future – but, I think a better use of the final chapter is to tell you what I think we (and the future Paramedics) need to succeed in whatever is coming down the road;

Ethics

Yes, it's true. I think we all would like to think that we are an ethical crowd and I think we are. The problem is that there are ethical questions now being asked that we never believed would be a part of our world; How long do we work a code before we call it and can we call it in the field at all? How early for a newborn do we have to do *everything?* When a patient shows us a DNR and it doesn't have the (fill in the blank) filled out, what do we do? After we have arrived to find a patient in their final moments and they tell us they don't want anything done, what do we do?

This does not include the many ethical questions that come up on the personnel operation side; I *earn* sick time, so why shouldn't I be able to take it anytime, even if I'm not sick? That's not *stealing*. I just need a *stress day*. I saw that medic give the wrong medication but I'm no rat – I'm not telling anyone. I need to get off on time so why can't I divert the Ambulance to the station on the way to the call? Its *only* three blocks difference.

Ethics is something I would like to think everyone has – and they do. However, we could use an occasional *sanity check* on our ethical dilemmas.

Balance

All of us work hard. Many of us, dinosaurs as we are (yes, I admit it), have *lived to work*. Some of us have the battle scars of such a work ethic – divorces, children who don't know us or who are mad because we seemed to spend more time at the firehouse or substation, than at home. We tried to make sense of that by telling ourselves we *liked* to be there because *they understood me*. The truth is that we simply didn't have enough balance in our life. We forgot that our family came first (I know we say it but do we practice it?) and lost them somewhere along the way. Sometimes, we lost ourselves, either through drugs or alcohol.

The bottom line is that we should always give 100% when we are working, but we should always remember to *work to live*.

We must – MUST – have balance in our lives. Get a hobby, one you enjoy and one that is, hopefully, away from patient care (a part time job on the BLS transport service isn't a hobby), go back to Church. Yes, I said go *back* - because I know what you do with that Sunday morning (I went to the "Church of the Sunday sleep-in" for years), Volunteer at a local animal shelter, start a book club, write a book, go sing in the local choir, learn to play an instrument, go hunting, camping, go discovering with your kids, your spouse or a best friend (NOT your partner). There are so many things that you can branch out in and, as we have said in this book, only a limited amount of time. If you want to change the world, take the world one corner at a time and don't choose a familiar corner. Always challenge yourself.

Never say never

No matter what it is you want to accomplish, be it school, marriage, a family or to ride a bicycle. Those who have sat in the "cheap seats" and told others, "You'll never do that" or, "We can't do that – we've never done that before" or, the famous "we've ALWAYS done in that way", are the life-suckers who drain the energy out of everyone's dreams. They are miserable in their life and, to make their world seem normal, must bring everyone down to their level.

It's sad but true.

I went back to school at the age of 43. I was the oldest in class but never gave up and actually had a fantastic time. I made friends with some really smart young people (and some really slow ones as well) and reached my dream of obtaining a college degree (from a Medical School, no less!). I have obtained my private pilot license, owned a single engine airplane, received my advanced open water scuba certificate, watched open heart surgery (live, in theatre), stood on the front lawn of the Taj Mahal (yes, the one in India) and never jumped out of a working airplane (hey, even I have my limits).

The point is that those who decide to accomplish one of their dreams, have no idea what they may bring in the future. Will it take a few years to do? So what? At the end of the adventure, the world will be open to you – maybe for the new adventure, maybe for the next challenge.

Those life-sucking negative people who choose not to take a chance? They'll be older. Period.

Decide which one you want to be and go after it!

Stop taking yourself so seriously

Yes, it's true that no matter how you try, the neighbors will know you as "the Paramedic" because they see you in your uniform more than in civilian clothes. Change that! Walk the dog, go biking, strike up a conversation, offer to help someone with their firewood. Realize that you are not a job, but a person.

That's particularly hard for us guys (and it may be for women as well) but it must be done. The sooner you realize that being humble beats being the King fills your heart with the kind of joy you can't find anywhere else.

Wake up every morning thankful for simple things

We work in a career that we see people's lives change in a second. They lose their ability to walk, to hear, to see or to enjoy life.

Every morning when I wake up, I thank God, for seeing and hearing that morning. It's the small things that we seem to forget.

I can walk without aid, have an occasional pain somewhere, but always feel great and realize another day is at hand. I probably have the same minor medical issues many of you have – but complaining about them to people doesn't make me feel any better and, generally, brings them down.

So, what about those of you who have those challenges? Maybe your health isn't the best. Maybe your hearing is shot or your eyes don't see as clear as they once did. You have pains that are, at times, horribly painful.

Someday, we will all see why some of us go through those trials – and it will all make sense. Until that day, God gives us the tools we need to do, what we need to do. It's our job to figure out what that is, and we can't do that if we sit around in bed, bemoaning our poor situation or wishing that *something* would change.

To everyone who has been a part of my life, whether in EMS or in my other life, thank you for helping me be the best person I can be.

Now, put this book down and go *do something fantastic!!*